WHAT THE EXPERTS ARE SAYING

"Dr. Avery has compiled a gem of a book integrating chemistry, biology and medical science with historical, social, legal and public policy considerations focusing on one of the most important issues of our day: the use of marijuana. The narrative is a beautifully written page-turner that brings medical science to life. Undergirded by the perspective of Christian faith, this volume is a uniquely valuable resource for healthcare professionals, decision-making bodies, church leaders and the public."

—*Robert M. Carey, MD, MACP, FRCP, FRCPI, FAHA*
Dean, Emeritus and Professor of Medicine, University of Virginia School of Medicine

---

"Dr. Avery has made a major contribution to the cannabis discussion in the U.S. with this book. His pragmatic approach is founded in and supported by good science and his prose easy and fun to read. This book is a must read for all who are curious about what the cannabis plant has become and where it is going. Even those who do not share Dr. Avery's Christian beliefs will gain a great deal from this book and those who do share his convictions will find great insight on that front. I highly recommend this book and am glad to have it on my shelf."

—*Ben Cort*
Speaker, author of **Weed, Inc.** *and CEO of The Foundry Steamboat Springs*

"This is a timely book which is easily read both lucid and informative plus a complete poem from George Herbert. The design features multiple clear subheadings, which makes it ideal for the busy physician, and includes clearly marked scriptural comments. It starts with history and includes chemistry, pharmacology and clinical descriptions with a good selection of endnotes. I found the discussion of the political intrusions into the functioning of the FDA and the classification of evidence from mere anecdotes to a few proper trials very helpful. Physicians will find the book very helpful as they attempt to pick up the bits from this ill-conceived experiment, and the general public will find the evidence they need to berate the politicians who caved in to the pressures from those who will make fortunes out of our children."

—*John Patrick, MD*
Physician, author and speaker on medical ethics, faith and public policy

---

"If you want to know the facts, rather than the fiction, on marijuana and CBD oil, this is the resource you need. It is well researched, it is shared in an easy to understand style and it is an essential tool to guide you, help your family and influence your community. Legalization of medical and recreational marijuana has swept across our country like a tsunami. For you and your family's safety, how do you separate facts from the fiction on this important issue? Read this great resource! You will be glad you did. It is like sitting down for a long talk with your doctor on this important issue. Is it marijuana harmless or a health hazard? Should it be legalized? What effect will it have on your community if it is legalized? For answers to these and many other questions, you need this book. I don't know of a better resource to recommend."

—*David Stevens, MD, MA (Ethics)*
Author, speaker and CEO Emeritus, Christian Medical & Dental Associations

MARIJUANA

AN HONEST LOOK AT THE WORLD'S MOST MISUNDERSTOOD WEED

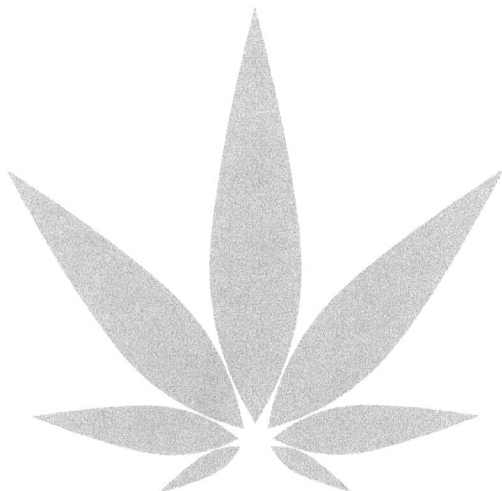

James Alan Avery, MD

The Christian Medical & Dental Associations was founded in 1931 and currently serves more than 19,000 members; coordinates a network of Christian healthcare professionals for personal and professional growth; sponsors student ministries in medical and dental schools; conducts overseas healthcare projects for underserved populations; addresses policies on healthcare, medical ethics and bioethical and human rights issues; distributes educational and inspirational resources; provides missionary healthcare professionals with continuing education resources; and conducts international academic exchange programs.

For more information:
Christian Medical & Dental Associations
P.O. Box 7500
Bristol, TN 37621-7500
888-230-2637
www.cmda.org • main@cmda.org

Cover design, interior layout and editing by Mandi Mooney.

ISBN 978-1-7344968-0-2

2020931094

Printed in the United States of America

To Jan

I would have accomplished little had you not been right by my side these past 38 years. All that I am proud of in my life, we have done together, with our Lord and Savior.

You and I have been an amazin' team—the '69 Mets have nothing on us.

This book took more time and energy than I had ever imagined, but you always understood, constantly adapted, endlessly edited and gave me grace at all times when I needed it.

Our daily walks, with ice cream cone in hand, and our four-mile runs by the river were always the best and most centering parts of my writing days.

By God's grace, we did this book hand-in-hand, arm-in arm.

Merci mon amour.
Je t'aime plus que la vie elle-même.

"Find a good spouse, you find a good life—and even more: the favor of God!"
—Proverbs 18:22, MSG

TABLE OF CONTENTS

FOREWORD

by Mike Chupp, MD, FACS

A few months ago, my wife Pam and I were sitting at our dining room table with our three young adult daughters, ages 18 to 24, when the topic of marijuana legalization came up. I wish I could say I was the one who brought it up, but I believe one of them asked, "Hey Dad, why wouldn't Christian doctors want marijuana made legal when it has so many benefits, like helping cancer patients and seizure patients?" The discussion that followed was lively (most of our family dinner table discussions are) and most revealing for my daughters. It was also revealing for me because my three daughters, who love the Lord and care about pleasing God and their parents, had been clearly influenced by the talking points of the marijuana industry and the "local representatives" of that industry.

I wish I had already read this book by Dr. James Avery about "the world's most misunderstood weed" before that conversation with my daughters. Dr. Avery's book comprehensively deals with the issues that have been so prominent in our national dialogue for the last several years, and he does so from the perspective of a seasoned hospice and palliative care physician. Recognized for his excellence in hospice and palliative care with numerous awards, he also has two amazing "in house" consultants on this subject: his sons, Dr. Jonathan Avery (Director of Addiction Psychiatry at Weil Cornell Medical College) and Joseph Avery (law school graduate and current PhD candidate at Princeton). Given Dr. Avery's background and recognized clinical expertise, he was asked by CMDA CEO Emeritus Dr. David Stevens to lead the efforts in developing CMDA's position statements on medical and recreational marijuana in 2018. You can find those position statements (which align very well with the information and perspectives in this book) in the appendix of this book or at *www.cmda.org/marijuana.*

I believe you will especially appreciate Dr. Avery's excellent summaries at the end of every chapter. Unique to this book are the Christian perspective sections at the end of multiple chapters, which are applicable to a biblical perspective on marijuana and its usage, as well as really any potentially abused substance, including alcohol. Each of these thoughtful, challenging perspectives could stand alone as material for a Bible study for non-medical groups or with students, residents or graduate healthcare professionals. You will want a copy of this book in your office or at home as a key reference tool when asked for your perspective by patients, parishioners, peers or the media. I don't think you'll find a better Christian treatise with more information about this controversial plant that God created than *Marijuana: An Honest Look at the World's Most Misunderstood Weed.*

The Focused Attention of Our Journey

"Honesty and transparency make you vulnerable. Be honest and transparent anyway."
—Mother Theresa

There is a passage from the book *Gilead* in which the narrator, Reverend John Ames, remarks, "This is an interesting planet. It deserves all the attention you can give it." This book is my attempt to give focused attention to one relatively inconsequential herb springing up from this orb we call earth.

Discussions about cannabis tend to generate robust opinions, passionate debates and heated arguments. Such "discussions" typically end up obscuring truth as each side "cherry-picks" from their preferred facts and doesn't acknowledge earnest considerations from the other side. Scientific realities and truths are lost in the superfluity of words and sardonic comments.

It is my goal in this book to help people separate fact from emotion, truth from myth. Americans are being asked to make substantial and sometimes personal choices regarding marijuana in their homes, in their workplaces, in their houses of worship and at the voting box. In this cultural moment, a dispassionate, objective and scientific view is desperately needed.

However, this book is the product of *my* journey, and personal blind spots and biases are unavoidable. So, a bit about my life journey—both professionally and personally.

I am a Visiting Assistant Professor at the University of Virginia, and I am board certified in hospice and palliative medicine, internal medicine and pulmonary. I am a Fellow in the American College of Physicians, the American College of Chest Physicians and the American Academy of Hospice and Palliative Medicine.

I come to this discussion with no hidden agendas. I have no financial stake in any marijuana stocks or companies. I have never had a family member hurt or helped by marijuana.

In my role as a hospice physician, prescribing psychoactive drugs has been an integral part of my professional life; in fact, I have written more prescriptions for opioids on some days than most physicians have written in a full year. The psychoactive characteristic of a drug is simply one factor I consider when prescribing or recommending a medication. I have no problem writing a prescription for a psychoactive medicine when I know it will bring more benefit than harm to a suffering patient.

The seeds for this book were planted about a year ago when I was asked to be on a medical committee exploring marijuana. What I found stunned me. At that time, I tended to be noncommittal regarding marijuana. A *laissez-faire* attitude characterized my response when some of my hospice patients informed me they were using marijuana.

But once I started reading the journal articles and the science research, I soon realized that the gap between the actual science and public perception was huge. Alex Berenson, former pharmaceutical investigative reporter for *The New York Times*, put it this way, "…in all my years as a journalist I had never seen a story where the gap between insider knowledge and outsider knowledge was so great, or the stakes so high."[1] The telos of this book is to bring science and reason into the discussion and narrow that gap.

> When it comes to marijuana, the gap between current scientific evidence of adverse consequences and public perception is large and increasing. The telos of this book is to bring science and reason back into the discussion.

It is also important for the reader to know that my Christian faith, I hope, permeates all I do and write. As I began writing this book, I came to the conclusion

I could not write about marijuana in a manner that ignores my deepest beliefs, experiences and commitments. I trust the reader will not be offended if I express my conviction that the Bible expresses truth about God and life.

This does not mean this book will be pointless for those of other religions or no faith. It simply means I want to be transparent and honest with you, and you deserve to know I have no hidden ambitions. In addition, I hope to state my deepest faith convictions with humility, politeness, generosity, tolerance and gentleness, fully knowing that unspeakable evils have been committed throughout the centuries—and are still being committed—by nominal Christians, often in the name of Christ.

Because I wrote this book with a sensitivity to all faiths and beliefs, I have placed Christian insights at the end of some chapters and have not integrated it with the main text. These sections, headlined with a green biblical icon, will express how I believe the Bible and the Christian faith address that chapter's content.

Finally, it seems to me that an interdisciplinary comprehensive look at marijuana through the lens of history, science, public policy and faith provides remarkably consistent, coherent and invaluable insights regarding the complex issues facing us concerning marijuana.

My hope is this approach will help all people to think more deeply, clearly and honestly about this vitally important issue of our day.

CITATION

1   Berenson, Alex, *Tell Your Children: The Truth About Marijuana, Mental Illness, and Violence*. Glencoe, Illinois: Free Press; 2018.

INTRODUCTION

L'herbe a Tous les Maux

(The plant against evil, pains and other bad things)

"History doesn't repeat itself, it rhymes."
—Mark Twain

More than 30 million people in the United States use it today. That's one of every seven adults. Can that many people be wrong? Most of these people will tell you quite readily that it calms them down, helps them feel relaxed and makes them more pleasant to be around. Some will say this over-the-counter preparation helps them with concentration and makes them more productive at home and at work. Many enjoy it so much they use it first thing in the morning and last thing at night. Mary Kate Olsen, Rihanna, Emily Blunt, Simon Cowell and Keira Knightley use it regularly.

Studies clearly show it acts as a strong appetite suppressant; the more it is used, the less hungry a person feels. Many people claim they no longer have any need of fad diets, as it helped them drop the necessary pounds. Researchers tell us it also increases the body's metabolism, increasing the energy and calories burned. Weight loss, they say, is inevitable. It will keep you lean and trim. It also raises your heart beat naturally—just like exercise—and that's a good thing. The heart is a muscle, and the more a muscle works, the stronger it gets.

And it is good for society. In 2016, tax revenues from its purchases amounted to more than $13.8 billion. Just think of the number of programs this natural plant provided: meals for hungry families, medical insurance for the poor, road construction, city developments, funds to senior centers, etc. More than 650,000 jobs depend on the growing, manufacturing and selling of this herb.

And let's not forget history. This herb has been used for thousands and thousands of years in South, Central and North America. It was considered by the natives to be a gift from the creator and was frequently the centerpiece of spiritual ceremonies. It was also considered a medicine and was given to those suffering from all kinds of ailments including colds, asthma, fatigue, headaches, tuberculosis and the aches of old age. It was considered so valuable that it was used as a form of currency and was often exchanged as a payment for goods.

On a sun-drenched morning in 1492, Christopher Columbus and his three ships landed somewhere in the Bahamas. While he planted the Spanish flag in the soil, the local inhabitants offered him this herb as a token of friendship. Considering this plant one of the treasures and wonders of the New World, Columbus brought it back to Europe. In his 1568 book *The New Found World*, Thomas Hacket described this plant in glowing terms: "There is another secret herb…which they most commonly bear about them, for that they esteem it marvelously profitable for many things…The Christians that do now inhabit there (have) become very desirous of this herb."

Almost immediately after its introduction by Columbus, the medicinal properties of the "New World Herb," as it was sometimes called, interested physicians all over Europe. More than a dozen medical texts were published touting this herb as a cure for everything from arthritis to epilepsy to influenza. "Anything that harms a man inwardly from his girdle upward might be removed by a moderate use of the herb," boasted a smitten physician. In 1560, Jean Nicot earned fame and fortune when he used the "New World Herb" to cure the incapacitating headaches of Catherine de Medicis, the Queen of France. Headlines followed, and the French ardently called it "l'herbe a tous les maux" (the plant against evil, pains and other bad things).

All across Western Europe, people were discovering and exploring its recreational uses. In Moliere's famous play *Don Juan*, the main character commends its virtues in the opening lines:

> *"…there is nothing like it. It's the passion of the virtuous man and whoever lives without it isn't worthy of living. Not only does it purge the human brain, but it also instructs the soul in virtue and one learns from it how to be a virtuous man. Haven't you noticed how well one treats another after taking it…it inspires feelings, honor and virtue in all those who take it."*

By 1565, the plant was becoming widely known as nicotaine, the source of its genus name today, *Nicotiana*. The chief commercial crop of the genus is *Nicotiana tabacum* or *N. tabacum*, which is known today as tobacco. If you thought I was discussing marijuana rather than tobacco, that is understandable. Mark Twain is purported to have said, "History doesn't repeat itself; it rhymes." And the history of tobacco certainly rhymes with the history of marijuana.

Maybe you view marijuana as being very different than tobacco, and *only* see it as a harmless, even healthy herb. One that provides a pleasant "high" making people creative, kind and mellow. If I am describing you, you will learn in this book that marijuana addiction is real and a risk at every age. You will understand the danger cannabis poses to adolescents, pregnant women, people predisposed to mental illness and society. And if you believe marijuana is a healthy panacea for many of the ailments and ills of life, like the now laughably outdated thinking about nicotine, you will see how politics, policy and accessibility have prevailed over medical science, exposing millions to fraudulent health claims and dangerous self-treatment. On the other hand, maybe you *only* think of marijuana as a poisonous plant, like tobacco, one that leads to physical illness. Or maybe you *only* see it as an evil drug that leads people into moral ruin or spiritual danger. Or perhaps you liken it to heroin and feel it should be outlawed from society entirely. If I am describing you, you will be surprised to know there are *potential* medical benefits to be drawn from the substances contained in the *Cannabis* plant; after all, there are already three FDA-approved prescription medications derived from *Cannabis*. And if you tend to stereotype all marijuana users as lazy and non-productive hedonists, you will better understand the Augean struggle of marijuana addiction, the stigma associated with it and how it typically commences in one's naïve and vulnerable teenage years.

This book is presented in five sections. The first section explores the history, botany, chemistry and biology of the *Cannabis* plant. The second section addresses the current state of *Cannabis: Vox Populi*, CBD, THC and the currently known health benefits and risks. The third section discusses FDA-approved medications, medical marijuana, recreational marijuana and decriminalization. The fourth section tackles the latest information about marijuana addiction, treatment and stigma. The fifth and final section scrutinizes 10 myths about marijuana. Each chapter will help us gain the knowledge, facts and information we need to grapple with the current issues we all face regarding marijuana in our homes, in our communities and at the voting booth. Although there is a logical order that enables a full picture, chapters do not depend on one another and can be read in any order. In an effort to make each chapter self-contained and whole, some material by necessity is repeated. Lastly, some chapters in the book will refer you to other chapters, so please feel free to skip around. But first, let's start our journey with botany since all of this fuss is just about a plant.

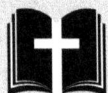

THE CHRISTIAN PERSPECTIVE
WISE, FAITHFUL AND RIGHTEOUS

Maybe you have only thought of marijuana as a "right" or "wrong" issue. When we look at Jesus' teaching parables in Matthew 25, we learn that our goal—our *telos*—should not be to merely do what is "right" rather than what is "wrong."

Christ's teachings, fully grasping the complexity of human realities and ethical dilemmas, prompts us to ponder deeply what is "wise" rather than "unwise" (Matthew 25:1-13: the parable of the 10 virgins). It pushes us to consider our identity and ask ourselves if we are being faithful servants or unfaithful servants (Matthew 25:14-31: the parable of the 10 talents). Finally, in Matthew 25:31-46 (the parable of the sheep and goats). Jesus asks us to consider ourselves as adopted sons and to behave in a way that is befitting such an undeserved righteous position.

As Christians, we should fully embrace the botany, history, chemistry, biology and intrinsic characteristics of marijuana and overlay the beauty rubric of what a wise daughter, faithful servant and righteous son might think and do. It's hard work, but it's worth it.

A PRAYER

Dear Father, help me to hunt down truth wherever it leads. Entrust me with wisdom, show me the way of Veritas. Grant me courage, fortitude and vigor to run full to the end and allow me to experience bounteous joy in this quest—this adventure—called life. May it all be to your glory.
Amen

It's Just a Plant...Or Is It?

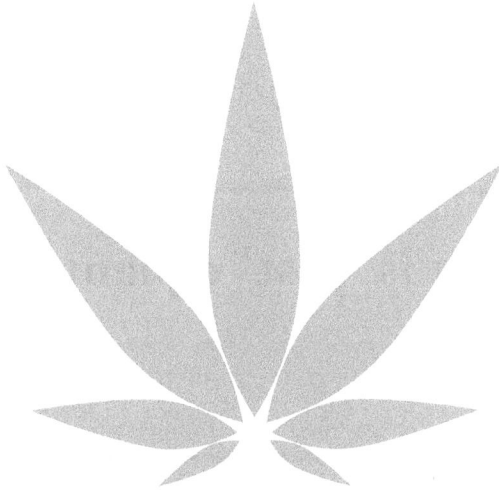

In a 2012 interview, Brad Pitt explained he was smoking marijuana to cope: "I got really sick of myself at the end of the 1990s...I was hiding out from the celebrity thing, I was smoking way too much dope, I was sitting on the couch and just turning into a doughnut and I really got irritated with myself."

Around that time, a trip to Morocco with Angelina Jolie precipitated a new awareness and determination. "I saw poverty to an extreme I had never witnessed before...and the children were inflicted with a lot of deformities...I just quit. I stopped grass then—I mean, pretty much—and decided to get off the couch."

"Oscar Nominee Brad Pitt On the Unmentionables:
Marriage, Politics and Religion"
The Hollywood Reporter
January 25, 2012

CHAPTER 1

Marijuana is "just" a plant...or is it?

"I think people need to be educated to the fact that marijuana is not a drug. Marijuana is an herb and a flower. God put it here. If He put it here and He wants it to grow, what gives the government the right to say that God is wrong?"
—Willie Nelson, singer, songwriter, musician

Marijuana—it's just a plant! Even though I will contradict those four words at the end of this chapter, they give us a firm foundation on which to begin our discussion about this fascinating herb. It's just a plant. Fortunately for us, botanists have conducted extensive research and studies on the *Cannabis* plant. Unfortunately, the nomenclature of the *Cannabis* plant is a bit confusing.

Cannabis is a genus of flowering annual plants in the Cannabaceae family indigenous to Eastern Asia. Within the genus *Cannabis*, there are three main species: *Cannabis sativa, Cannabis indica* and *Cannabis ruderalis*. However, most people simply refer to the entire genus as *Cannabis sativa* since many botanists believe *Cannabis indica* and *Cannabis ruderalis* are a subspecies of *Cannabis sativa* (or *C. sativa*). In addition, crossbreeding of these three strains has led to more than 6,000 hybridized strains and using the term *C. sativa* to describe all *Cannabis* plants almost became a necessity for non-botanists.

Cannabis sativa plants can be further categorized based on the cultivating practices. Hemp is *C. sativa* plants cultivated for fiber and seed production, while marijuana is *C. sativa* plants cultivated for recreational and medicinal use. Therefore, marijuana and hemp are simply different expressions of the species *Cannabis*, but they are worlds apart in function and use.

Before we proceed, let's clarify the terms we are using. When someone properly uses the word *Cannabis*—italicized and capitalized—or an italicized capital "*C*" with a period, they are using the scientific term for the genus *Cannabis* and are referring to hemp and/or marijuana. Therefore, *Cannabis*, *Cannabis sativa* and *C. sativa* can be used interchangeably. The word cannabis—non-italicized and non-capitalized—is the common name for marijuana and is synonymous with marijuana, weed, hashish, Mary Jane and a host of other colorful names.

Terms	Significance of Name	Refers to	Part of Speech	Synonyms
Cannabis (capitalized and italicized)	Scientific name for the entire genus	Hemp or Marijuana	Noun	*Cannabis sativa* *C. sativa*
cannabis (non-capitalized and non-italicized)	Common name for marijuana	Marijuana only	Noun or adjective	Marijuana, Weed, Pot, Hashish, Mary Jane

HEMP

The Hemp plant is typically found in the Northern Hemisphere and was an extremely common crop in Europe for centuries as it was grown for textiles, rope and feed. Archaeologists tell us it was spun into usable fiber 10,000 years ago.

Even today, there is a significant worldwide market for hemp as it is refined into an amazing variety of commercial items including paper, textiles, clothing, biodegradable plastics, paint, insulation, soap, biofuel, food and animal feed. Canada, Australia, Austria, China and Great Britain are the most important agricultural producers of hemp.

Hemp has low concentrations of tetrahydrocannabinol (THC), the active psychoactive ingredient in marijuana. The legality of industrial hemp varies between countries. In the United States, hemp must have less than 0.3% THC on a dry weight basis.[1] Therefore, hemp has no psychoactive or hallucinogenic properties. Despite being in the same genus, botanists tell us it is relatively easy to differentiate hemp from marijuana as it has little branching and can grow up to 13 feet tall.

MARIJUANA

In contrast, the marijuana plant is grown worldwide. It has a branching structure and is generally less than six feet tall; in fact, it can be as short as two feet. It is grown mainly for the THC in the dried flowers and subtending leaves of the female cannabis plant, and these create the stock material from which all other preparations are derived. THC levels in the marijuana plant range widely between 3% and 30%. A "joint" is simply the dried flowers and subtending leaves rolled in paper and smoked like a cigarette. A "bud" is a specific part of the dried cannabis flower that people like to smoke because it is especially potent.

The stem, stalk, pistils, roots and seeds have little to no THC. Interestingly, the big leaves with its many leaflets (the universal image of marijuana) have very low levels of THC and are typically thrown out after the plant is trimmed.

Cannabis Sativa	Branching	Maximum Height	Uses	THC
Hemp	Few	13 feet	Feed Cordage Textiles	Less than 0.3%
Marijuana	Many	Two to six feet	Medicinal Recreational	3% to 30%

PLANT BREEDING

Plant breeding is the science of altering the qualities of a plant in order to produce desired properties. Scientists, entrepreneurs, investors and farmers are pouring money into marijuana research to create plants that meet the demands of consumers for a faster and more intense high. Powerful lights, genetic engineering, shortened growth cycles and special soils have created a "new marijuana," which are plants with extremely high THC levels and some achieving levels 20 times higher than the marijuana of the 1960s.[2,3]

MARIJUANA PREPARATIONS

Cannabis-derived products may contain any chemical from the marijuana plant, but THC products dominate the multi-billion-dollar market. From the stock material (dried flowers and subtending leaves), many preparations, products and extracts can be derived, and some of these are nearly pure THC. For instance, you can get THC concentrates over 90% at practically every Colorado marijuana dispensary.[4]

- **Kief** is a powder sifted from the leaves and flowers of cannabis (marijuana) plants. It can be consumed in powder form or compressed to produce cakes of hashish. In some areas of the country, the term kief is used interchangeably with marijuana.
- **Hashish** is a concentrated resin produced from pressed kief. It is consumed

orally, smoked or vaporized ("vaped").

- **Hash oil** is a potent resinous matrix of cannabinoids obtained by solvent extraction. It is formed into viscous oil or mass, similar in appearance to honey or butter. Hash oil is often considered the most powerful of cannabis products because of its high THC concentrations. Marijuana enthusiasts will sometimes refer to hash oil as "710," which is "OIL" upside down, marijuana concentrate, extract, shatter, wax, honey oil (BHO), budder and taffy.
- **Tinctures** of THC and other cannabinoids can be extracted from the *Cannabis* plant matter using high-proof alcohol. This formulation allows for precise dosing, typically with an eyedropper. High potency tinctures of THC are often referred to as "green dragon."
- **Infusions** of innovative preparations are formed when *Cannabis* plant material is mixed with various solvents and then pressed and filtered. Examples of solvents include cocoa butter, dairy butter, cooking oil, glycerin and skin moisturizers. Depending on the solvent, these may be used in cannabis foods (edibles) or applied topically.

Because of the plethora of names associated with marijuana, its products and other paraphernalia, a glossary is included in the appendix of this book.

As you can see from the various cannabis goods I have described, the issues around marijuana are not about a plant; instead, they are about the production and commercialization of an intoxicant, THC. In other words, most of the cannabis being consumed today is not marijuana—the real product is THC. But I am getting ahead of my story....

KEY POINTS

Cannabis is an annual herbaceous flowering plant indigenous to Eastern Asia. It has been bred for use in industry (hemp), as an intoxicant (marijuana) and for medicinal purposes (both hemp and marijuana). Most strains of the plant have been bred to produce tetrahydrocannabinol (THC), the principal psychoactive constituent. The dried flowers and subtending leaves are the most widely consumed form and create the stock material from which all other cannabis preparations are derived.

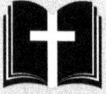

THE CHRISTIAN PERSPECTIVE
IT'S NOT "JUST" A PLANT

"In the beginning, God created Cannabis sativa. And God saw that it was good."
—Genesis 1, Avery Revised Standard

My tongue-in-cheek restating of Genesis, although humorous, illustrates some key points. As Christians, we believe the story of Genesis that God created everything: man, cows, watermelons and marijuana. It was all declared good.

"And God said, 'Let the earth sprout vegetation, plants yielding seed, and fruit trees bearing fruit in which is their seed, each according to its kind, on the earth.' And it was so. The earth brought forth vegetation, plants yielding seed according to their own kinds, and trees bearing fruit in which is their seed, each according to its kind. And God saw that it was good. And there was evening and there was morning, the third day."
—Genesis 1:11-13, ESV

It was all declared good throughout Genesis 1. But, "the fall" happened, sin entered the world and man began using creation for selfish, unethical and unprincipled purposes. For example, fire is good. It keeps us warm at night, but countless homes, businesses and lives have been lost to arson. So, we need to add a qualifier to the word "good." Everything is "good" for its *intended purpose*. Since the Bible tells us that humans were given dominion over all the earth and told to subdue it, our mandate is to use everything our Creator gives us to its fullest potential and greatest intended good—to God's glory. But even this sentence is inadequate as it fails to describe the allurement inherent in the mysteries and excesses in creation. I believe science defines life in ways that are too small.

For instance, marijuana is not "just" a plant. In the same vein, the birth of a baby is not "just" the beginning of life for another fetus. A kiss is not "just" two lips touching each other. The death of a beloved spouse is not "just" the cessation of the heart muscle. Marilyn Robinson said it well in *Gilead*, when she wrote that people sometimes use the word "just" when they "want to call attention to a thing existing in excess of itself."

According to the Christian faith, everything is more than it seems, and our noble mandate as created beings is to embrace the "excess" and "mystery" radically fundamental to everything. "Embracing the excess" means seeing and using things beyond the material. It means having a view of life that results in "God-pleasing choices"—good choices and wise choices, with the belief that every decision, whether momentous or trifling, has eternal significance. In *On Friendship*, Cicero says with deep conviction that wisdom and goodness are one. And, ultimately, being wise and doing good is our challenge with *Cannabis*…and with everything in life.

A PRAYER

O Lord God, who inhabits all time, the universe is your footrest, the stars declare your splendor and majesty. The earth and everything in it, the herbs and plants of the field, all of this is yours. Wisdom and goodness are undeserved gifts from your storehouse. Be generous to us with your blessings: enlighten our eyes that we can see the wonders of this world, increase our faith that we discern the mysteries of your creation and your handiwork in everything.
Amen

CITATIONS

1   *https://nifa.usda.gov/industrial-hemp*
2   National Academies of Sciences Engineering and Medicine. The Health Effects of Cannabis and Cannabinoids: The Current State of Evidence and Recommendations for Research. Washington, DC: The National Academies Press; 2017.
3   National Institute on Drug Abuse. Marijuana. July 2019. Accessed 9.01.19 at *https://www.drugabuse.gov/marijuana*
4   Alzghari SK et al, "To Dab or Not to Dab. Rising Concerns Regarding the Toxicity of Cannabis Concentrates," *Cureus* 2017 9(9),e1676.

CHAPTER 2

It's "Just" an Assembly of Chemicals

Two men walk into a bar. The first man orders H2O.
The second says, "I'll have H2O, too." The second man dies.
Chemistry jokes can be tricky.
I once told a chemistry joke and there was no reaction.

I f you are not laughing, this chapter is for you because you clearly are not a chemistry aficionado. (Full disclosure: I was a chemistry major and find chemistry jokes to be hilarious). The marijuana plant comprises more than 400 chemicals, of which more than 100 are cannabinoids, that is, chemicals unique to the *Cannabis* plant. Some experts have separated cannabinoids into the major cannabinoids (THC and CBD) and the minor cannabinoids (THC-V, CBN, THC-A, CBG and more than 100 others.) Even though all of these compounds together contribute to the unique pharmacological properties of cannabis, THC dominates the clinical picture because it is by far the most prevalent and psychoactive cannabinoid.[1]

THE MINOR CANNABINOIDS
Minor cannabinoids have a variety of pharmacological effects (some are psychoactive and others are not), but their concentrations are low and only contribute in a secondary way to the overall clinical effect. However, almost all marijuana users

will tell you the potency of any batch of marijuana is not totally dependent on the THC concentration. This probably reflects the cumulative effect of the minor cannabinoids in that particular plant. You can expect to hear more about these minor cannabinoids over time as researchers are currently isolating, concentrating and studying many of them.

THE MAJOR CANNABINOIDS

1. **THC or delta 9-tetrahydrocannabinol (▲9_THC):** THC is the chemical responsible for most of marijuana's psychological effects. It is the most psychoactive cannabinoid and the one primarily responsible for the euphoria or high.

2. **CBD or cannabidiol:** In contrast to THC, CBD is not psychoactive, and it actually lessens or counteracts the high associated with THC. CBD products constitute a small portion of the cannabis commercial market but may have medicinal potential.

In this chapter, I'm going to focus on what happens chemically when THC is consumed as it is the substance that governs the effect when it comes to marijuana. CBD, because of the closeness of the chemical formula, is similarly metabolized and excreted, but activates different receptors.

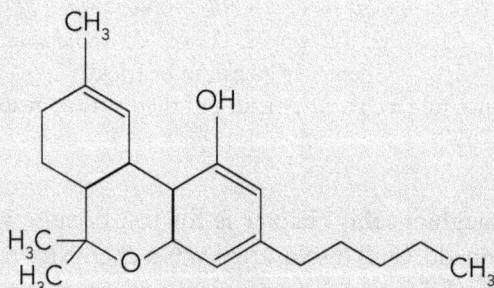

Tetrahydrocannabinol (THC)

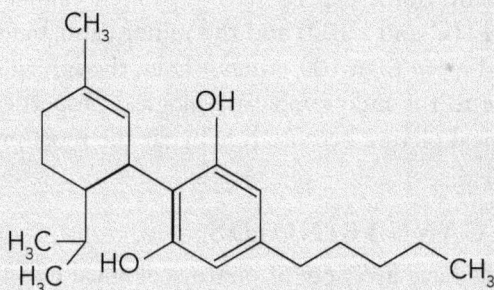

Cannabidiol (CBD)

MARIJUANA POTENCY

Since THC is, by far, the most psychoactive cannabinoid, the potency of marijuana is best estimated by the percentage of THC (see sidebar #1). Older Americans remember marijuana as a relatively weak psychotropic drug, and they are right. In the 1970s, most marijuana contained less than 2% THC.

A study that analyzed samples from pot seized by the U.S. Drug Enforcement Administration (DEA) from 1995 to 2014 also showed an increase in potency of "illicit cannabis plant material" from 4% THC content in 1995 to 12% in 2014.[2,3] Today, marijuana testing facilities are reporting average THC concentrations between 10 and 30%, with more potent strains being created every year to meet demands from users for a faster and more intense high.[4] Comparing the marijuana of the 1970s and 1980s with the marijuana of today is like comparing a beer to grain alcohol.

Does a THC percentage of 30% mean 30% of the weight of a marijuana plant is pure THC?

The short answer is no. Scientists use a process called "gas chromatography" and it measures with great precision the percentage of the THC available in a dry sample selected.

The key here is a dry sample. Most marijuana plants contain plenty of water and other fluids, so the percentage of THC is not the percent by weight of a marijuana plant you see growing in a field.

The percentage of THC is a very useful tool for tracking the efficiency of farming and estimating the potency of a marijuana plant.

SMOKE, INHALE OR VAPE

While the majority of the THC is delivered to the smoker, about 30% is lost to pyrolysis.[1] When smoked, inhaled or vaped, THC is rapidly absorbed through the alveoli of the lungs and into the bloodstream. Alveoli are the tiny air sacs that allow for the passage of oxygen, carbon dioxide and other gases, like THC. Millions of alveoli are in the human lung, and if they were all cut open and laid flat, they would create a surface area roughly one-third the size of a tennis court, yielding an amazingly efficient and rapid absorption system.

Therefore, THC is rapidly absorbed and can be detectable in the blood within seconds of the first puff, typically reaching peak blood concentrations within three to 10 minutes (average eight minutes).[5,6] This produces a rapid high and is the reason most marijuana consumers, despite the well-known hazards, still prefer smoking, vaping or inhalation.

ORAL INGESTION

The absorption of THC into the blood after oral ingestion is relatively slow compared to smoking. When taken orally—either as an oil, tincture, capsule or edible—the liver metabolizes some of the THC as it passes from the intestines into the general bloodstream, slowing and reducing the blood levels of THC. Generally, it takes 30 to 90 minutes to start feeling the effects. THC reaches peak blood levels about one to three hours after ingestion, with the peak level lasting longer compared to smoking or vaping. Compared with smoking, oral ingestion diminishes the initial high but prolongs its duration.

Edibles are of particular concern to emergency room physicians because numerous people, unaware of the delayed onset, get impatient for an effect and take another edible thinking "the first one didn't work." Sadly, they sometimes end up in a hospital emergency room with a THC overdose (see chapter 20). Edibles made up a small percent of total cannabis sales in Colorado yet a much larger percent of emergency room visits.

PASSIVE SMOKING

While the majority of the THC is delivered to the smoker, about 20% is released into the air. Although uncommon, studies have demonstrated conclusively that it is possible to test positive for THC just by being in close proximity to a smoker. The amount of THC absorbed depends on the environment (closed room versus a well-ventilated space), the duration of the exposure and the percentage of THC in the marijuana smoked.

ONCE IN THE BLOODSTREAM

Once in the bloodstream, THC rapidly distributes throughout the body. THC is lipophilic (fat-loving), which is the single most important physical property affecting potency, distribution and elimination. Because of its lipophilicity, THC leaves the bloodstream within three to four hours and penetrates into tissues with a high fat content, such as the liver, spleen, kidney, adipose and brain. THC also passes into breast milk, the placenta and the circulation of unborn babies.

Marijuana causes tachycardia (elevated heart rate) for up to three hours after smoking. An elevated heart rate may increase the risk of a heart attack, especially in the elderly and those with heart problems.

THC AND THE BRAIN

Once in the brain, THC attaches to cannabinoid receptors associated with thinking, decision-making, memory, pleasure, coordination, appetite and time perception. THC has other effects on the brain by releasing dopamine and interfering with information processing in the hippocampus, the part of the brain responsible for forming new memories.

The effects on thinking, memory, pleasure, coordination, appetite and time perception are what constitute the high or euphoria from marijuana, making it a popular and addictive drug. The high generally lasts about two hours, but coordination problems and impaired motor skills last another hour or so. This prolonged effect on motor skills (after the perceived high has ended and the user feels back to normal) probably contributes to the fact that marijuana is the second-most common psychoactive substance found in fatal car accidents.

The Blood Brain Barrier and THC

In the early 1900s, a bacteriologist named Paul Ehrlich was injecting dyes into the veins of animals. To his surprise, some of his dyes stained all of the organs except the brain. Intrigued by this finding, further studies by other scientists demonstrated the existence of a barrier between the body's blood circulation and the blood circulation in the brain.

What they discovered is a remarkable part of the human body called the blood-brain barrier, a semipermeable border that separates the circulating blood from the brain. This barrier works amazingly well protecting the brain from infections and other chemicals, which is why infections of the brain are rare when compared with other organs.

Lipophilic chemicals, however, like THC, pass easily and quickly through the blood-brain barrier and into the brain.

HIGHER DOSES OF THC GIVE MORE THAN JUST A LONGER AND GREATER HIGH

Higher doses of THC result, as expected, in longer and greater physical and mental effects than lower doses of THC. In addition, the psychoactive effects seen with higher doses of cannabis on an individual are often different and more worrisome than the effects from a lower dose, which suggests stimulation of additional areas of the brain. A dose-related psychosis, increased psychiatric illnesses and higher addiction rates[7] are some of the reasons committees in the Netherlands, Uruguay and Colorado are advocating that marijuana containing greater than 15% THC be classified as a "hard drug."[8] Furthermore, with increased use, "desensitization" occurs, resulting in the need for higher doses to achieve the same euphoric effect. The full range of adverse effects from higher dose THC has not been well studied.

THE ELIMINATION OF THC FROM THE BODY

Because THC is lipophilic, it is not eager to leave fatty tissues. Over days and weeks, it slowly leaks out from fatty tissues back into the blood stream where it is eliminated through feces and urine. Because of the concentration in fatty tissues and the slow release, cannabis has a half-life in humans of about two months.

MEASUREMENT OF THC IN THE BODY

An accurate measurement of THC in the body is becoming more important as it is critical for pharmacokinetic studies, drug treatment, workplace drug testing and drug impaired driving investigations. Cannabinoids can be detected in saliva, blood, urine, hair and nails using various analytical techniques.

Urine is the preferred sample because it can be easily obtained, contains a higher concentration of THC metabolites and has an extended detection time. Immunoassay is the preliminary screening method in drug testing programs. However, false negative and false positive results occur from structurally-related drugs and artifacts such as adulterants affecting pH, detergents and other surfactants. For this reason, any positive result using immunoassay should be confirmed by chromatographic techniques.[1]

A one-time user of marijuana will usually "pass" a THC urine test within a few days after stopping. A person who only consumes THC on the weekends will typically pass a THC urine test within a few weeks after that last joint. A regular

---

Cannabinoid Receptors

THC is the "psychoactive" ingredient, responsible for the euphoria or high that comes from marijuana due to its partial agonist activity on type-1 cannabinoid receptors (CB1).

CB1 receptors are found in the brain in high concentrations as well as in the gastrointestinal tract and skeletal muscle. THC's chemical structure is similar to the endogenous cannabinoids (specifically anandamide), which are neurotransmitters that bind to CB1.

These cannabinoid receptors are critical for brain development, particularly the formation of brain circuits used for decision-making, attitude/mood formation and stress response. Some of the most serious side effects in the young brain (those under 25 years of age) are related to the effect of cannabis on these receptors. CBD has low affinity for CB1 and CB2 receptors, and that is the reason it is not psychoactive.

user (i.e., daily or almost daily) will generally pass a THC urine test after a month or two. However, all of these are estimates as the elimination of THC from the body depends on the individual's fat content, liver function, exercise levels, kidney function and individual metabolism.[9,10,11]

Because of the long half-life, it is difficult to determine whether a positive urine for THC represents recent drug use or continued excretion of residual drug from a day, a week or a month ago. Therefore, it is currently impossible to definitely establish that a driver is impaired from marijuana based on a THC test. Algorithmic models have been advanced in an attempt to determine whether THC levels represent recent use, but these have not been found to be accurate.

KEY POINTS

The marijuana plant contains more than 100 cannabinoids. These can be sub-grouped into the "major cannabinoids" (THC and CBD) and the "minor cannabinoids." Even though all of these compounds together contribute to the unique properties of any particular plant, THC dominates the clinical picture because it is by far the most prevalent and the most psychoactive cannabinoid.

The absorption of THC depends on the manner in which it is consumed. When smoked or vaporized, THC is rapidly absorbed and can be detected in the blood within seconds. Oral consumption results in a much slower absorption. THC is highly lipophilic ("fat-loving") and, therefore, passes easily into the brain, placenta, breast milk and adipose tissues.

The psychoactive effects seen with high THC concentrations are often different than the effects experienced from lower concentrations suggesting the stimulation of additional areas of the brain. The physical and mental effects from high-dose THC are especially worrisome, and early studies suggest higher rates of addiction and increases in acute psychoses, paranoia and other psychiatric illnesses.

Because cannabinoids are excreted slowly, they stay in the body for weeks. Scientists have not been able to develop a method to determine whether a positive urine for THC represents recent drug use or continued excretion of residual drug from a day, a week or a month ago.

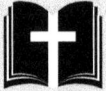

THE CHRISTIAN PERSPECTIVE
SCIENCE AND FAITH

This might be a good place to discuss my view regarding science and faith. The Bible is an eclectic diverse compilation of history, law, moral teachings, poetry, prophecy, songs, parables, letters, law, theology, rituals, etc. But, please note, there are no chapters on chemistry or biology or physics, as the Bible is not a scientific text.

Yet, Christians have often taken the lead in developing the principles of science. Motivated to know God, they believe studying and understanding His creation will bring insight into the divine. After all, you can tell much about an artist by examining his oeuvre. For instance, is the Earth "just" a spinning cooling cinder as the result of a massive Big Bang explosion? Or is it covered with the fingerprints of God?

Throughout history and right up to our modern age, there have been leading scientists who fully grasped science and fully embraced faith (see below). If they lived today, I believe all would say the earth eventuated from the Big Bang and the earth is inundated with the handiwork of the divine.

Frances Bacon (1561 – 1624) is credited by most historians with the development of the scientific method. He stressed observation, repetition and verification rather than philosophical speculation. He established the Royal Society of London, a group of scientists, philosophers and physicians who met regularly to discuss and debate the pressing issues of the age. Like many devout Christians, he believed God gave us two "books" to study: the Bible and nature. He once said, "There was never law, or sect, or opinion did so much magnify goodness, as the Christian religion doth."

Johann Kepler (1571 – 1630) is considered by most to be the founder of astronomy. He discovered the laws of planetary motion, established the principles behind celestial movements, conclusively demonstrated the heliocentricity of the solar system and contributed to the development of calculus. Kepler also coined the phrase, that scientific research and discovery was "thinking God's thoughts after Him," a maxim adopted by numerous Christian scientists and researchers.

Blaise Pascal (1623 – 1662) was a mathematician, physicist and inventor. He developed the first calculator, vigorously defended the scientific method and broke scientific ground in the study of fluids, geometry, probability and pressure. And he just as forcefully defended the Christian faith in many of his letters, public speeches and his book *Pensées*. He wrote in *Pensées*, "There are two kinds of people one can call reasonable: those who serve God with all their heart because they know him, and those who seek him with all their heart because they do not know him." In France today, Blaise Pascal Chairs are awarded to outstanding international scientists.

Isaac Newton (1642 – 1727) is credited with discovering the Law of Gravity and the three laws of universal motion, and he stressed calculus as a critical branch of mathematics. Newton wrote in defense of the Christian faith and, specifically, against atheism. He penned in *The Principia*, "This most beautiful system of the sun, planets and comets, could only proceed from the counsel and dominion of an intelligent and powerful Being."

Louis Pasteur (1822 – 1895) was famous for developing the germ theory of disease and vaccines, and he made other significant contributions to the fields of chemistry and physics. Pasteur also helped to disprove the theory of the spontaneous generation of life. Many consider Pasteur to be the greatest biologist who ever lived. His famous quote describes the depth of his belief: "Little science takes you away from God but more of it takes you to Him."

Francis Collins (1950 –) is a physician-geneticist who discovered the genes associated with a number of diseases and led the Human Genome Project. He is currently the director of the National Institutes of Health (NIH) in the United States. Collins is also a prolific author, writing a number of books on science and religion including *The Language of God: A Scientist Presents Evidence for Belief*. He founded and serves as president of The BioLogos Foundation, which promotes discourse on the relationship between science and religion, saying, "The God of the Bible is also the God of the genome. He can be worshipped in the cathedral or in the laboratory. His creation is majestic, awesome, intricate, and beautiful," as he wrote in *The Language of God*.

Justin L. Barrett (1971 –) is an experimental psychologist and Director of the Thrive Center for Human Development and Professor of Psychology at Fuller Graduate School of Psychology. A former researcher at Oxford, Barrett is a cognitive scientist and, in 2011, published a widely respected book entitled *Cognitive Science, Religion, and Theology*. Barrett was described in the

New York Times as "an observant Christian who believes in 'an all-knowing, all-powerful, perfectly good God who brought the universe into being,' as he wrote in an e-mail message. 'I believe that the purpose for people is to love God and love each other.'"[12]

All this to say that there have been and there are countless scientists who see no conflict between their faith in God and their scientific research. In fact, most of these scientists believe we can only understand our universe fully when we view everything in light of the biblical narrative.

It has been my experience that science, the Bible and the Christian faith are mutually supportive and intellectually consistent. I believe devout Christian believers are obligated by the Christian virtues of integrity and fidelity to pursue scientific truth wherever it leads—even when it might rub church authorities and scientific organizations the wrong way. Kepler and Galileo would be good examples of scientists who kept their faith *and* their scientific beliefs even in the face of harassment by the church and other scientists.

Following in their esteemed footsteps, we will proceed with truth and science wholeheartedly in this book, not just when it suits our argument or purposes. I believe my Christian faith and the Bible demand that.

A PRAYER

Dear Creator God, I seek to learn more about you and your creation. But your ways are as high above mine as Alpha Centauri is above the earth. I am insignificant and doltish in comparison. But you told us to ask for wisdom and to knock for understanding. Respect, awe and submission are the beginning of wisdom. Help me to place my mind and will under yours. Thank you for being the underpinning and foundation of science. Grant me wisdom to see your artistry in everything. Open my eyes to see the genius, orderliness, love, truth and beauty of your creation and your sacrifice on the cross. For yours is the kingdom, the power and the glory forever.
Amen

CITATIONS

1   Sharma P, Murthy P et al, "Chemistry, Metabolism, and Toxicity of Cannabis: Clinical Implications," *Iranian Journal of Psychiatry* 2012;7(4):149-156.

2   National Institute on Drug Abuse. Marijuana. July 2019. Accessed 9.01.19 at *https://www.drugabuse.gov/marijuana*

3   ElSohly MA, "Changes in Cannabis Potency Over the Last 2 Decades (1995-2014): Analysis of Current Data in the United States," *Biol Psychiatry* 2016;79(7):613-9.

4   *https://www.cnn.com/2016/10/21/health/colorado-marijuana-potency-above-national-average/index.html*

5   Law B et al., "Forensic aspects of the metabolism and excretion of cannabinoids following oral ingestion of cannabis resin," *J Pharm Pharmacology* 1984;36:289-294.

6   Owens SM et al., "1251 radioimmunoassay of delta-9tetrahydrocannabinol in blood and plasma with a solid-phase second-antibody separation method," *Clin Chem* 1981;27:619-624.

7   Arterberry BJ et al., "Higher average potency across the United States is associated with progression to first cannabis use disorder symptom," *Drug Alcohol Depend* 2018; 195:186-192.

8   European Monitoring Centre for Drugs and Drug Addiction. Netherlands Country Drug Report 2017. Luxembourg: Publications Office of the European Union; 2017.

9   Smith-Kielland A, Skuterud B et al., "Urinary excretion of 11-nor-9-carboxyΔ9-tetrahydrocannabinol and cannabinoids in frequent and infrequent drug users," *Journal of Analytical Toxicology* 1999;23(9), 323-332.

10 Reiter A, Hake J, Meissner, C et al., "Time of drug elimination in chronic drug abusers: Case study of 52 patients in a 'low-step' detoxification ward." *Forensic Science International* 2001;119, 248-253.

11 Niedbala RS, Kardos KW et al., "Detection of marijuana use by oral fluid and urine analysis following single-dose administration of smoked and oral marijuana," *Journal of Analytical Toxicology* 2001;25(7/8), 289-303.

12 Justin Barrett. *New York Times* Darwin's God March 4, 2007.

CHAPTER 3

The History of *Cannabis*

"One must wait until evening
To see how splendid the day has been."
—Sophocles

Popular history is often distorted, and this has certainly been the case with marijuana. There are several reasons for this: we love anecdotal stories, over-generalizations and conspiracy theories. We tend to value story over expert historical analysis, and there have been plenty of anecdotal stories about marijuana's benefits and harms throughout the years. But rarely is the history of anything as unambiguous as stories and anecdotes suggest. Another significant problem is our tendency to think in generalities. For instance, marijuana has been called "an evil weed" and, by others, "God's perfect gift to mankind." This happens because people make aeonian judgments from just a few facts.

History is often flawed by our love of conspiracies. Countless major events in history—the life of Jesus, the Kennedy assassination, the Moon landing and September 11—have been questioned by conspiracy theorists who warn of powerful secret groups that control all the world's levers. Marijuana advocates and detractors have hundreds of conspiracies regarding marijuana.

Despite the brevity of this chapter, I have studiously avoided anecdotes, over-generalizations and conspiracy theories. I have tried my best to present an accurate history by only including solid historical events or, when those are lacking, stating clearly when a certain event is simply believed, speculated or debated.

INDIA (2000 TO 1000 BC)

Cannabis sativa, this unique annual plant, has been a food, clothing, medicine and psychoactive agent for thousands of years. *Cannabis* is believed to have originated in the mountainous regions north of the Himalayas in India.

The natural levels of THC and CBD in a typical *Cannabis* plant were most likely very low. Since CBD lessens the psychoactive effects of THC, *Cannabis* in its original state was probably a mild sedative or calming agent. One of the ancient Sanskrit Vedi poems from India (2000 to 1000 years BC) celebrated the *Cannabis* plant as one of "five kingdoms of herbs…which release us from anxiety."

EGYPT AND CHINA (1700 BC TO 500 BC)

Cannabis found its way to Egypt, in its naturally low THC form, and it is mentioned in at least three ancient medical texts: Ramesseum III Papyrus (1700 BC), Eber's Papyrus (1600 BC) and the Berlin Papyrus (1300 BC). However, it appears the *Cannabis* plant found its main use in the manufacturing of rope, clothing, paper and sails. Its seeds were used as feed for animals and for human consumption. Interestingly, burned cannabis seeds were found in China and Siberia in the graves of shamans (500 BC).

MIDDLE EAST AND ISLAM (700 AD)

After a period where little about *Cannabis* is known, the story picks up in the 700s AD when hashish enters the picture again. Because hashish is concentrated and smoked, this may represent the first time we truly have a THC-rich cannabis (i.e., marijuana), although this is intensely debated. Hashish spread throughout the Middle East and into parts of Asia, Africa and Europe after about 800 AD, which corresponded with the spread of Islam. Early Muslim jurists differentiated cannabis from alcohol. While Islamic restrictions on alcohol remained strictly enforced, cannabis use was prevalent in the Islamic world until the 18th century. Indeed, hashish is mentioned in a sunny light-hearted manner in the story "The Tale of the Hashish Eater" in the Arabian and Islamic classic *One Thousand and One Nights*. Today, most Islamic scholars and religious authorities declare marijuana as *haram*

"I drink not from more joy in wine nor to scoff at faith – no, only to forget myself for a moment, that only do I want of intoxication, that alone."
—The Rubaiyat of Omar Khayyam

(or religiously forbidden), citing the *hadith* (an Arabic term meaning report or saying) of Muhammad that says, "If much intoxicates, then even a little is *haram*."[1]

THE NEW WORLD (1545 TO 1700 AD)

Cannabis crossed the Atlantic Ocean not long after Columbus, arriving in the New World around 1545 AD when the Spaniards introduced it into Chile. Because *Cannabis* is a fast-growing and easy-to-cultivate plant with many uses (especially in textiles and rope), it was widely grown throughout Spanish missions in the Southwest and colonial America.

In the early 1600s, farmers in the Virginia, Massachusetts and Connecticut colonies were required to grow hemp as it was considered an essential plant for survival. These plants had low levels of tetrahydrocannabinol (THC), and it doesn't appear that the mild anti-anxiety or sedating effects of cannabis were widely known, if at all.[2]

I'm sorry to disappoint some marijuana history buffs who seem to love to spread myths, but George Washington and Thomas Jefferson grew hemp, not marijuana.

RECOMMENDED BY PHARMACIES AND PHYSICIANS (1800s AD)

In the 1830s, Sir William Brooke O'Shaughnessy, a physician studying in India, found that *Cannabis* extracts helped patients suffering from cholera. It reduced abdominal pain (probably spastic colon), nausea and vomiting. By the late 1800s, *Cannabis* extracts found their way to pharmacies and physicians' offices throughout the United States, and they were used to treat stomach problems and other general ailments.

PROHIBITION (1900s)

During the 20th century, alcoholism, social disintegration of the family, homelessness and corruption prompted people across the globe to speculate that society's ills might be mitigated by prohibiting psychoactive substances—including alcohol and marijuana. In 1911, Egypt prohibited hashish. Between 1914 and 1919, laws were passed in Russia, Norway, Iceland and Finland prohibiting alcohol. And, in 1920, citizens in the United States approved a nationwide constitutional ban on the production, importation, transportation and sale of all alcoholic beverages, including beer and wine.

Cannabis also attracted attention in the United States. In the early 1900s, Mexico went through a violent and bloody revolution. Thousands of Mexicans fled to the United States, and with them came their long-standing practice of smoking marijuana. Deprived of alcohol, Americans along the southern border seemed especially receptive.

However, unemployment during the Great Depression created fierce competition for jobs and stoked resentment against immigrants. In the Southeast and other regions, this sparked a backlash against Mexican immigrants and Mexican products. This overt racism led to a public denouncement of the "evil Mexican weed." This headline in *The Richmond Times-Dispatch* from March 9, 1913 gives the prevailing sentiment: "Evil Mexican Plants That Drive You Insane."

As a result, and consistent with the Prohibition era's view of all intoxicants, 29 states outlawed *Cannabis* by 1931. In 1937, under the newly formed Federal Bureau of Narcotics (FBN), *Cannabis* became a banned substance in the entire country. The Marijuana Tax Act of 1937 was the first federal law to criminalize marijuana nationwide. The act imposed an excise tax on the sale, possession and transfer of all marijuana and hemp products, and it effectively criminalized all but industrial uses of the plant.[3]

58-year-old farmer Samuel Caldwell was one of the first people prosecuted, convicted and sentenced to prison under the act. He was arrested for selling marijuana on October 2, 1937, one day after the act's passage. Caldwell was sentenced to four years of hard labor.[4] During World War II, hemp prohibitions were lifted as the government needed hemp cloth for the war effort (tents, coverings, clothing for the troops, etc.) After the war, when hemp was no longer needed, the Air Force and Marines were ordered to destroy all remaining crops.

MODERN CHEMISTRY, *CANNABIS* AND THC (1960 TO 2020)

In the 1960s, things changed significantly for *Cannabis* as a new scientific invention, called Nuclear Magnetic Resonance (NMR) spectroscopy, allowed chemists to better identify, purify and study the ingredients in various substances. The molecular structure of THC was discovered in 1964 at the Hebrew University of Jerusalem by organic chemist Raphael Mechoulam and his associates.[5] Soon thereafter, other scientists discovered that THC was the source of cannabis' psychoactive properties. For the first time, there was great interest in isolating, purifying and studying THC.

Slowly, at first, THC levels began to rise in marijuana plants. Scientists, entrepreneurs, investors and farmers poured money into marijuana research creating the "new marijuana" we have today. Powerful lights, genetic engineering, shortened growth cycles and special soils yielded plants with extremely high THC levels, with some achieving levels 10 to 20 times higher than the marijuana of the 1960s.

THE WAR ON DRUGS IN THE UNITED STATES (1970s AND 1980s)

As part of the "War on Drugs," President Richard Nixon signed the Controlled

Substances Act of 1970, listing marijuana as a Schedule I drug—along with heroin, LSD and ecstasy— thereby classifying marijuana as a "drug with no medical uses and a high potential for abuse." This severely hindered federal funding sources for research. Two years later, the National Commission on Marijuana and Drug Abuse released a monograph entitled, "Marijuana: A Signal of Misunderstanding." This report, know as the Shafer Commission report, recommended the lowering of penalties for possession of small amounts of marijuana and limited prohibition. Most government officials ignored the findings and recommendations.

TOLERANCE REIGNS IN THE NETHERLANDS

In the 1970s, the Dutch went a different direction in creating a market for marijuana. The Netherlands Dutch Ministry of Justice applied a *gedoogbeleid* (tolerance policy) toward "soft drug" use and, even though there were no significant changes to the laws, marijuana was essentially decriminalized.

Almost immediately, the infamous Dutch "cannabis coffee shops" began springing up. The term "drug tourism" originated in the Netherlands as people traveled from other countries with the sole intention of purchasing or using marijuana. By the 1990s, the number of coffee shops in the country had grown to 1,500, and the average concentration of THC in the cannabis sold in coffee shops had increased from 9% in 1998 to 18% in 2005.[6]

Alarmed by the rising THC levels, a Dutch government committee report recommended that cannabis with more than 15% THC be labeled as a hard drug, putting it into the same category as heroin and LSD. Legislation has been proposed, but the recommendation has yet to be implemented. If implemented, the sale of 15% or higher THC would not be permitted in the Netherlands.[7]

Surprisingly, the "War on Drugs" in the United States and *gedoogbeleid* in the Netherlands resulted in similar results, as marijuana became the most commonly used illicit drug in both countries.

MEDICAL MARIJUANA GAINS APPROVAL IN THE UNITED STATES

In February 1979, in an article that appeared in Emory University's *The Emory Wheel*, head of pro-legalization group the National Organization for the Reform of Marijuana Laws Keith Stroup said, "Medical Marijuana is a red herring to help usher in legalized marijuana." A total of 17 years later, despite a dearth of medical evidence, California became the first state to legalize medical marijuana. Initially, the law restricted access to marijuana to those with severe chronic or terminal illnesses.

A confluence of politics, profits, celebrity endorsements, cannabis enthusiasts and influential lobbyists managed to get medical marijuana laws approved in several states. Numerous pro-marijuana state campaigns were lavishly financed by billionaire George Soros's Drug Policy Alliance (DPA) and other lobby groups, often overwhelming the cadre of volunteers opposing these laws. As of October 2019, Washington, D.C., 33 states and the U.S. territories of Guam and Puerto Rico allow the use of cannabis for medical purposes.

In June 2018, the residents of Oklahoma voted in favor of legalizing medical marijuana, and officials estimated about 80,000 patients (2% of the population) would register in the first year to be eligible for medical marijuana. One year later, more than 3.5% of the entire population of the state had registered, easily surpassing all predictions. According to news reports, people came out in droves to apply for licenses because (like several other states) Oklahoma's medical cannabis law lacked a list of qualifying medical conditions a patient must prove to enroll.[8] Thus, a patient could get medical marijuana without the need for any medical diagnosis.

RECREATIONAL MARIJUANA GAINS APPROVAL IN THE UNITED STATES

Stroup's words were prescient: medical marijuana laws served as a convenient stepping stone for the legalization of recreational marijuana. Every state that has legalized recreational marijuana legalized medical marijuana first.

In 2012, Colorado and Washington became the first states to legalize cannabis for recreational use. As of September 2019, nine more states and Washington, D.C. have followed suit. In these states, you can find THC in breath sprays, brownies, sodas, hot cocoa, hard candies, cakes, candy bars, gummy bears, coffee, ice cream, cotton candy and the list goes on and on.

THE TIDE MAY BE TURNING

In 2018, Arterbury and colleagues recommended that policy makers in the United States consider instituting an upper limit of THC because of the addiction potential of high-potency marijuana. According to the authors of the study, Uruguay and the Netherlands, two countries known for freewheeling drug policies, are contemplating similar limits.[9]

The rollback of cigarette use began with then Surgeon General Luther Terry's bold warnings in 1964. In August 2019, Surgeon General of the United States Jerome Adams, MD, paralleled Dr. Terry by issuing a warning to Americans about the health dangers of marijuana, stating unequivocally in an interview that medical marijuana is not medicine and warning about its use by teens, young people and women during pregnancy.

ONE MUST WAIT UNTIL EVENING...

Of course, the history of marijuana is still being written. Will the current rush to legalize marijuana result in another epidemic like the opioid crisis? Or will new wonder drugs evolve from the chemicals in the *Cannabis* plant reducing the sufferings of many?

More books will be written, and more analysis will be done, but one must wait until evening...until the last page is written...to know if the day was splendid or not. But, for now, let's focus on what we know because it is only noon.

> "One must wait until evening
> To see how splendid the day has been."
> —Sophocles

KEY POINTS

Historically, marijuana was most likely a mild sedative until 700 AD when the technique to develop hashish oil became available. THC levels remained low until the 1960s when chemists for the first time identified THC as the main psychoactive ingredient. Since the 1990s, THC levels have risen dramatically as investments in farming and chemical technology yielded a THC-rich high-potency marijuana never imagined in the 1960s.

At the same time, cannabis promoters in the last 20 years strategically reinvented marijuana as a "medicine" instead of a "hallucinogenic intoxicant," thereby transforming the discussion. A confluence of politics, profits, cannabis enthusiasts, celebrity endorsements and highly paid lobbyists influenced public opinion, and medical marijuana laws were approved in numerous states. This has served as a strategic stepping stone to the legalization of recreational marijuana.

CITATIONS

1   From the book *Practical Laws of Islam* by Sayyid Ali Hosseini Khamenei (published by CreateSpace Independent Publishing Platform:2014): "Question 1392: What is the ruling in the matter of using narcotics, such as hashish, opium, heroin, morphine, and marijuana, be it by way of eating, drinking, smoking, injecting or applying them anally? And what is the view on selling, buying, and dealing in them in general, i.e., carrying, transporting, storing, or smuggling? Answer: It is haram [religiously forbidden] to use narcotics in any way because it results in considerable adverse effects in terms of personal health and social cost. By the same token, it is haram to deal in narcotics in any way, i.e., carrying, transporting, storing, selling, buying, etc."

2   *https://www.history.com/.amp/topics/crime/history-of-marijuana*

3   This act was overturned in 1969 in *Leary v. United States* and was repealed by Congress the next year.

4   *https://norml.org/aboutmarijuana/the-first-pot-pow*

5   Mechoulam R., "Marihuana chemistry," *Science* 1970; 168: 1159– 66.

6   *https://enacademic.com/dic.nsf/enwiki/12855*

7   European Monitoring Centre for Drugs and Drug Addiction. Netherlands Country Drug Report 2017. Luxembourg: Publications Office of the European Union; 2017.

8   *https://www.tulsaworld.com/news/local/marijuana/one-year-after-sq-vote-oklahoma-near-no-for-patients/article_7ba3a964-39cb-51d1-98b3-082eaa388c74.html*

9   Arterberry BJ et al., "Higher average potency across the United States is associated with progression to first cannabis use disorder symptom," *Drug Alcohol Depend* 2018; 195:186-192.

Cannabis in the Year 2020

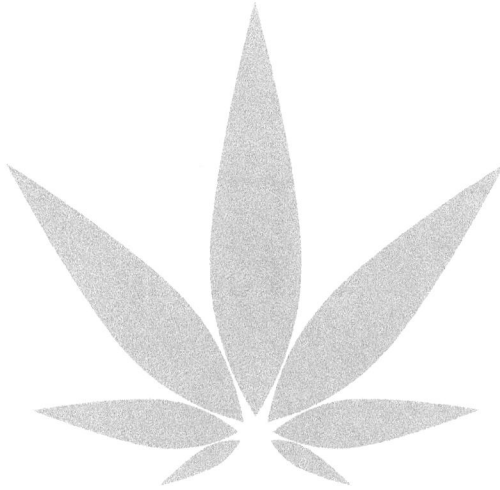

"I had motives for not wanting the world to have a meaning;
consequently assumed it had none, and was able without any
difficulty to find gratifying reasons for this assumption."
—Aldous Huxley, *Ends and Means*

The robust, almost inevitable tendency for humans to rational-
ize and justify our desires and predictions is legendary. Huxley
went on to say, "Most ignorance is vincible (conquerable). We
don't know because we don't want to know. It is our will that de-
cides how and upon what subjects we shall use our intelligence."

Whether you want to know or not, in the next four chapters, we
will discuss the current state of CBD and THC, as well as the
benefits and risks associated with marijuana. Ponder Huxley's
words as you read Section 2.

Il n'y a pas plus sourd que celui qui ne veut pas entendre.

CHAPTER 4

Vox Populi

Nec audiendi qui solent dicere, Vox populi, vox Dei,
quum tumultuositas vulgi semper insaniae proxima sit.

(Don't listen to those who keep saying the voice of the people is the voice of God,
since the riotousness of the crowd is always very close to madness.)
—A letter from Alcuin to Charlemagne in 798

"What is truth?" asked Pilate to Christ and perhaps himself (John 18:38, ESV). The only response was a deafening silence. Some believe truth is simply what the majority thinks it is. If so, this could have been a Lilliputian book because public opinion is remarkably consistent in viewing marijuana as a natural, safe and harmless substance. Oscar Wilde could have been describing marijuana proponents when he famously said, "Public opinion…is an attempt to organize the ignorance of the community, and to elevate it to the dignity of physical force."

A huge shift in conventional wisdom occurred in the last 20 years, even though most Americans do not use marijuana. In fact, only 15% used it even once in 2017.[1] However, Gallup organization's latest polls showed that almost two in every three Americans favor legalizing marijuana.[2] At the same time, large studies in peer-reviewed medical and scientific journals have turned far more negative toward cannabis as associated health risks have become more evident and worrisome.[3]

Americans' Support for Legalizing Marijuana Continues to Rise

Do you think the use of marijuana should be made legal, or not?

■ % Yes, legal

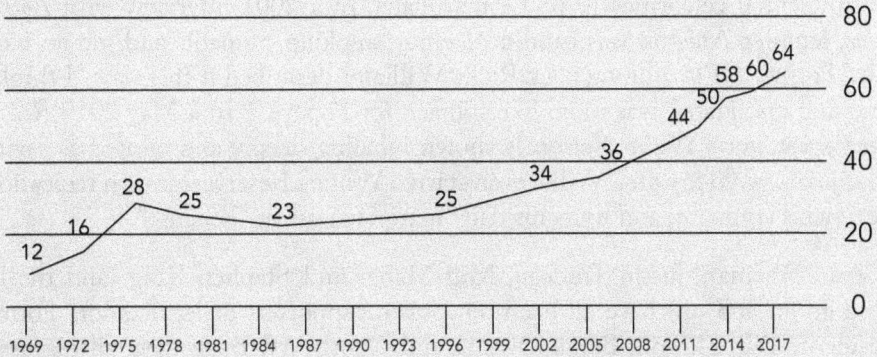

80

64
58 60
50
44
60

36
34
40

28
25
25
23
20

16
12
0

1969 1972 1975 1978 1981 1984 1987 1990 1993 1996 1999 2002 2005 2008 2011 2014 2017

Graph information released by Gallup in October 25, 2017.

Just when you thought it was impossible for Republicans and Democrats to agree about anything, marijuana came to the rescue. In 2018, both Democratic Senator Minority Leader Chuck Schumer and former Republican Speaker of the House John Boehner expressed almost identical sentiments:

> "My thinking—as well as the general population's views—on the issue has evolved, and so I believe there's no better time than the present to get this done (legalization of marijuana). It's simply the right thing to do."
> —Chuck Schumer[4]

> "Over the last 10 to 15 years, the American people's attitudes have changed dramatically (towards legalization); I find myself in that same position."
> —John Boehner[5]

Mr. Boehner's change of heart was followed by an announcement that he was joining the advisory board of a large for-profit cannabis corporation named Acreage Holdings.[2] His compensation for this position was not stated, but evidently it was enough to also induce former Governor of Massachusetts Bill Weld to join his Republican colleague on the board.

These days, proposals to legalize medical or recreational marijuana are as likely to come from a Republican as a Democrat. Sometimes I feel Arnold Glasgow was describing our politicians when he said, "The fewer the facts, the stronger the opinion."

The legalization of recreational marijuana in Colorado in 2012 led many popular and influential celebrities to praise marijuana. In a 2001 interview with *Rolling Stone*, Jennifer Aniston was candid: "I enjoy smoking cannabis and see no harm in it." Former NFL running back Ricky Williams described it this way: "I think it (smoking marijuana) was more like spinach for Popeye."[6] In a May 2019 *Rolling Stone* cover story, Willie Nelson is shown inhaling deeply and quoted as saying, "Marijuana saved my life." Willie even started Willie's Reserve, his own recreational cannabis company, and touts his daily marijuana use as "healing."

Morgan Freeman, Justin Trudeau, Mill Maher and Stephen King (and the list could go on and on) have all been outspoken supporters of legalization. Former Presidents Bill Clinton, Barak Obama and George W. Bush have all discussed their use of marijuana—usually on late night talk shows—and typically with the host and everyone in the audience chuckling.

Even physicians are culpable. Almost half of oncologists (46%) say they had recently recommended medical marijuana to a patient, although more than half (56%) confessed they did not have sufficient knowledge to do so.[7]

In a review of medical cannabis in the December 2018 edition of *Mayo Clinic Proceedings*, the authors stated, "Public opinion and policy changes are rapidly transforming the landscape of U.S. cannabis consumption, frequently in the absence of scientific indications for which it is being promulgated."[8]

The logical next question is this: how did this happen? How has the consensus gentium moved so far ahead of science and reason? As I researched that question, the answer became obvious.

Money.

Patrick Kennedy, son of the late Senator Ted Kennedy and a former U.S. Representative in his own right, put it this way, "Many marijuana advocates have one goal in mind: to get rich."[9]

Despite disturbing scientific evidence, marijuana is becoming more and more normalized due to an aggressive marketing campaign. Powerful corporations and wealthy lobbyists have worked hard to reduce the public's perceived risk as they seek to commercialize marijuana and reap profits. And, as we have seen in states where it is legal, business owners have launched innovative and creative products to lure new and heavy users (i.e., customers). In his book *People of the Lie*, Scott Peck explains how "responsibility becomes diffused within groups so much that in larger groups it may become nonexistent…and our institutions become absolutely faceless. Soulless."

"Consider the large corporation," asks Peck. "Even the Chairman of the Board will say, 'My actions may not seem entirely ethical, but after all, they're not really a matter of my prerogative. I must be responsive to the stockholders, you know.'" Attitudes like that abound in marijuana businesses and even worry proponents of medical marijuana. In a *USA Today* article from August 21, 2019, Dr. Jordan Tishler, president of the Association of Cannabis Specialists and an advocate for legalizing medical marijuana, said, "There's an industry out there that wants to sell a lot of marijuana-based products regardless of whether it is safe or good for anybody."

Politicians have been especially disappointing in their lack of leadership and their dearth of interest in the science of marijuana. Many joined the marijuana bandwagon eagerly while wanting (and needing) additional tax revenues. In states where marijuana is legal, we've created perverse incentives whereby it is in the state's interest to encourage cannabis use in order to fill empty tax coffers. In the state of Washington, politicians gloated over the fact that they racked up $82 million in tax revenue in the first year of legalization.

Gandhi's Version of the Seven Deadly Sins

"Politics without principle, Wealth without work, Commerce without morality, Pleasure without conscience, Education without character, Science without humanity, Worship without sacrifice."

Endorsements by cannabis enthusiasts, non-profits and some celebrities have added to the chorus heard by the public, but it's all about money. Sadly, in America, "profits over people" is not an unknown concept or rare practice. We remember when Purdue Pharma pled guilty in 2007 to criminal charges of fraudulently marketing OxyContin (an addictive opioid medicine) and was fined $600 million in fines and penalties. The company's fine was trivial compared to its profits; it was just the cost of doing business. Even in late 2019, as Purdue flirts with bankruptcy, corporate executives are enjoying lavish retirements.

As asserted in a *New York Times* "opinion" article on January 4, 2019, well-funded marijuana advocates "shrewdly recast marijuana as a medicine rather than an intoxicant." This ploy ended up being more effective than their previous and more honest argument: personal freedom ("people should be allowed to do anything they want as long as it doesn't hurt anyone else"). The article went on to say that while they were promoting the positive medical aspects, they willfully ignored the risks:

"Legalization advocates have squelched discussion of the serious mental health risks of marijuana and THC."

The concerted effort to reduce risk awareness has definitely affected the average person on the street. Just look at the increasing number of pregnant women using marijuana. One hospital in Pueblo, Colorado reported that nearly half the newborns tested were positive for marijuana. "I believe it's beneficial. I don't think it is toxic in any shape or form," said a pregnant mom when interviewed by a Colorado TV station.[10]

Today's culture has made it almost impossible to discuss marijuana rationally. Anyone who raises even reasonable reservations about marijuana is derided as a Neanderthal, closet teetotaler or believer in "Reefer Madness." We need to objectively and rationally discuss the potential benefits and threats cannabis poses to individuals, families, society and the environment. As Gregory Hays wrote in his introduction to *Meditations* (Marcus Aurelius), "Our duty is to exercise stringent control over the faculty of perception, with the aim of protecting our mind from error."[11]

KEY POINTS

The *vox populi* says marijuana is a natural, safe and harmless herb.

Contrary to scientific realities, this sentiment has been swayed by celebrity endorsements, powerful and wealthy lobbyists, corporations seeking profits, politicians wanting tax revenues and cannabis enthusiasts espousing personal freedom.

This has resulted in a serious knowledge gap between popular belief and scientific reality.

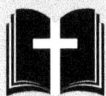

THE CHRISTIAN PERSPECTIVE
CAREFULLY CONSIDER THE OPINION OF THE MAJORITY

From the first pages of the Bible to the last, every reader is warned to beware the opinion of the majority. The first half of the Bible is replete with stories of prophets who lost their lives because they said things rulers and the majority did not want to hear. In the second half, we see the majority of religious leaders being blind to truth and influencing public opinion to such an extent that the public demanded the death of an innocent man, a man they had praised only days before.

History tells a similar story to the biblical narrative: the opinion of the majority is not necessarily the best assessment. At one point in history, slavery was thought to be perfectly fine by most people. In the 1700s, bloodletting was the preferred medical treatment. More likely than not, people 100 years from now will look at our time and exclaim, "How could they have believed that!"

"For the wisdom of this world is foolishness in God's sight...'The Lord knows that the thoughts of the wise are futile'" (1 Corinthians 3:19-20, NIV 1984). The truth of 1 Corinthians should give all of us pause whenever we read the latest poll or hear about the most popular movie. A belief that the majority tends to be right is probably enhanced in the United States because of our foundational belief in democracy. Any historian can burn up days and weeks recounting the political failures of democracies. After all, Germany was a democracy when it elected Adolf Hitler.

And carefully evaluate your own emotions. Discussions about marijuana can often get heated and passionate. Philosopher Jean-Jacques Rousseau argued that "feelings" will bring you closer to "the truth" than will reason. The Bible, however, warns us about following our heart (core emotions), while, at the same time, acknowledging that emotions are a gift from our Creator. Who of us hasn't had our emotions lead us astray at some time? Jeremiah 17:9 says, "The heart is deceitful above all things and beyond cure. Who can understand it?" (NIV 1984).

So much of what we read and hear is simply the majority's opinion or personal feelings. We must strive to see things as they are. The Bible calls us to be humble and vigilant in our search for truth and to live circumspectly and perceptively while carefully watching, questioning and challenging the opinion of the majority and our own emotions.

A PRAYER

Heavenly Father, you are the maker and sustainer of all things. You hold the keys to truth and wisdom. We are naturally disposed to our own fears, smallness and prejudices. Our desires, proclivities and predilections push us to ignoble places. Enlighten the eyes of our heart that we may see ourselves, others and the world clearly. May we have your eyes for a day, an hour, a moment? Help us to love what you love. Because that would change everything.
Amen

CITATIONS

1   Salomeh Keyhani S, Steigerwald S et al., "Risks and Benefits of Marijuana Use: A National Survey of U.S. Adults," *Ann Intern Med* 2018; 169(5):282-290.
2   *https://news.gallup.com/poll/225017/news-marijuana-legalization.aspx*
3   Berenson, Alex, Tell Your Children: *The Truth About Marijuana, Mental Illness, and Violence.* Glencoe, Illinois: Free Press; 2018.
4   *https://www.cnbc.com/2018/04/20/chuck-schumer-announces-plan-to-decriminalize-marijuana.html*
5   *https://www.bloomberg.com/news/articles/2018-04-11/ex-speaker-john-boehner-joins-marijuana-firm-s-advisory-board*
6   Kyle Newport, "Ricky Williams Compares Marijuana Use to 'Spinach for Popeye,'" Bleacher Report, last modified October 8, 2013.
7   Braun IM, et al., "Medical Oncologists' Beliefs, Practices, and Knowledge Regarding Marijuana Used Therapeutically: A Nationally Representative Survey Study," *J Clin Oncol* 2018; 36(19): 1957-62.
8   Ebbert J et al., "Medical Cannabis," *Mayo Clinic Proceedings* 2018; 93(12):1842-1847.
9   Kennedy P, Sabet K, "Don't let Big Marijuana prioritize profits over public safety," *Washington Post*, March 8, 2017.
10 *https://denver.cbslocal.com/2016/07/11/marijuana-pregnant-thc-positive-babies-colorado/*
11 Aurelius M, *Meditations*, New York: Modern Library; 2002.

CHAPTER 5

The Current State of
Cannabidiol – CBD

"Why that CBD Oil you bought is probably useless."
—*Chicago Tribune* headline, August 2, 2019

C annabidiol (CBD) is one of more than 100 unique compounds (i.e., cannabinoids) found in the *Cannabis* plant, and it has played second fiddle to THC, its psychoactive cousin. But CBD is no slouch as annual sales of CBD products in the United States have now exceeded $200 million and one estimate has the CBD market reaching $2.1 billion by 2020.[1]

CBD AS A MIRACLE COMPOUND

CBD is currently being marketed as a "cure-all for everything," and that is not hyperbole. According to manufacturers and advertisers, there is hardly a disease out there that won't benefit from adding CBD. Enthusiasts tout an amazingly broad range of healing powers and claim benefit in diabetes, cancer, pain, sleep, anxiety disorders and arthritis. And, yes, CBD has even made its way into dog treats.[2] Other promoters advertise it as the perfect "after-work relaxant" and the ideal supplement for enhancing sports performance. As we shall see, these claims have little or no basis in science.

THE MARKETING NARRATIVE

Here is the marketing narrative that has captured Americans: "CBD is safe, natural, has a broad range of healing properties and will give you all of the health benefits of marijuana without the psychoactive element." This powerful narrative has increased consumer demand and energized cannabis enthusiasts, farmers, investors and state governments.

Tony Spurrill, a chiropractor in Minnesota and vocal advocate for CBD, put it this way: "Hemp-based CBD oil is not the same as marijuana. You get the anti-inflammatory effects and the pain relief without the high. For some people, it really is and has been a lifesaver."[3]

LOW COST + PLENTIFUL SUPPLY = PROFIT

The other side of demand is "supply," and plenty of CBD is available as it can be isolated from both marijuana and hemp. The 2018 Farm Bill removed hemp (*Cannabis* with THC levels below 0.3%) from the list of controlled substances, and many farmers, anticipating the demand for CBD, in the United States began replacing corn, soybeans and tobacco with hemp.

These entrepreneurial farmers created a pipeline of inexpensive CBD that helped fuel an ever-expanding array of CBD products. Walk into any store that sells vitamins and supplements and you will see store shelves featuring CBD oils, gummy candies, honey, joint balms, capsules, creams and other products. CBD infused juices, sodas, coffee and beers are even becoming available in numerous locations. My local newspaper advertises a CBD product regularly.[4] Unfortunately, most of the people buying these products are wasting their money and might even be risking their health.

WHY THAT CBD OIL YOU BOUGHT IS PROBABLY USE-LESS (AND POTENTIALLY HARMFUL)

An August 2, 2019 headline in the *Chicago Tribune* summarized the truth regarding CBD accurately: "Why that CBD Oil you bought is probably useless." Because there is currently no effective regulation and monitoring of supplements in the United States, there is no way a consumer can guarantee a CBD product contains what is written on the label. In fact, concentrations of CBD have been found to be all over the map with little correlation to the advertised content. A November 2017 study published in *JAMA* found that 70% of CBD products were either over-labeled or under-labeled.[5] Marcel Bonn-Miller, PhD, the lead author of the study, believes irresponsible behavior by manufacturers and lax oversight by the states are responsible for the poor quality of many, perhaps most, CBD products.

"The big problem, with this being something that is not federally legal, is that the needed quality assurance oversight from the Food and Drug Administration is not available. There are currently no standards for producing, testing or labeling these oils," Dr. Bonn-Miller said. "So, right now, if you buy a Hershey bar, you know it has been checked over; you know how many calories are in it, you know it has chocolate as an ingredient, you know how much chocolate is in there. Selling these oils without oversight, there is no way to know what is actually in the bottle. It's crazy to have less oversight and information about a product being widely used for medicinal purposes, especially in very ill children, than a Hershey bar."[6]

The urgency to meet consumer demand and the lack of regulatory oversight has resulted in a large number of manufacturers (both ethical and unethical) hurriedly churning out products.

A contaminant, probably a synthetic cannabinoid, caused 52 poisonings in Utah in late 2017 and early 2018.[7] A study at Virginia Commonwealth University found cough suppressants and a dangerous synthetic in a different manufacturer's CBD products.[8]

Randomized Controlled Trial

A randomized controlled trial (RCT) is a type of medical experiment that has the goal of reducing bias when testing a new treatment or medicine.

This is accomplished by randomly allocating subjects to two or more groups, treating them differently and then comparing the results. One group—the experimental group, for example—would receive CBD, while the other—called the control group—would receive a placebo.

The two groups would then be monitored to see how effective the CBD was in comparison to the placebo.

RCTs are ideally blinded: information that may influence the participants or observers is withheld until after the experiment is complete.

RCTs reduce selection, allocation, observer and subject biases. A well-blinded RCT is considered the gold standard for clinical trials.

A SHOCKING LACK OF EVIDENCE

Despite consumer acceptance and rising sales, the evidence for CBD's health benefits is shockingly sparse. There is some preliminary evidence of benefit in a few human studies, but these are rare and hard to come by. The National Academies of Science, Engineering and Medicine (NASEM) in 2017 concluded that there was weak (or limited) evidence that CBD reduced anxiety symptoms as assessed by a public speaking test.[9]

As an anti-inflammatory, antioxidant and possible central nervous system depressant, there is great hope that CBD will *someday* be helpful in combating human disease and suffering. However, the type of preliminary evidence we currently have (by any objective standard) would absolutely require a randomized control trial (see sidebar) before CBD could ever be recommended by a reasonable healthcare professional.

SAFETY CONCERNS

Besides the scarcity of evidence, researchers and physicians have raised concerns regarding the safety of CBD. Clinical studies conducted for Epidiolex, an FDA-approved CBD medication, give us insight into the potential side effects of CBD. At a dosage of 20 mg/kg/day, side effects from Epidiolex have included diarrhea (20%), somnolence (25%), decreased appetite (22%) and increased levels of liver enzymes (16%). In addition, decreases in hemoglobin and hematocrit levels (anemia) and increases in serum creatinine (kidney function) have been reported.[10]

No data are available on the use of CBD in pregnant women. In animal studies, administration of CBD resulted in developmental toxicity, embryofetal mortality, decreased fetal body weight and structural variations. There are no data on the presence of CBD or its metabolites in breast milk or on its effects on the breast-fed infant or milk production.[10]

In December 2018, worried about the lack of studies and known adverse effects, the

---

Drug Interactions of CBD[9]

CBD is metabolized by CYP3A4, CYP2C19 UGT1A7, UGT1A9 and UGT2B7. Concurrent administration of moderate or strong CYP3A4 or CYP2C19 inhibitors can increase CBD serum concentrations and the risk of adverse effects.

CBD is a potential inhibitor of UGT1A9, UGT2B7, CYP2C8, CYP2C9 and CYP2C19. CBD may induce and/or inhibit CYP1A2 and CYP2B6; dosage adjustments of drugs metabolized by these enzymes may be needed.

Concurrent use of central nervous system depressants, including alcohol, may increase the risk of sedation and somnolence. CBD may also interact with other medications, such as blood thinners.

FDA stated unequivocally that CBD cannot be legally sold in either supplements or foods.[11] Because the FDA has only enforced their proclamation with warning letters (not fines) and because consumer demand remains high, many manufacturers have ignored the FDA and continue to promote and sell CBD products.

In 2013, a different over-the-counter dietary supplement (not CBD) began to become popular for sports enhancement. Tragically, this supplement caused a serious hepatitis outbreak leading to dozens of hospitalizations, two liver transplants and one death.[12] Given the large number of people taking CBD, physicians and public health officials are clearly worried something similar could happen with CBD supplements. After all, we already know it has caused an elevation of liver enzymes in clinical trials.

AN FDA-APPROVED CBD MEDICINE

In 2018, the FDA approved Epidiolex, a pharmaceutical-grade prescription CBD to treat intractable seizures in children with two rare syndromes: Lennox-Gastaut (LGS) and the Draver syndrome. (We will discuss this medication in more detail in Chapter 8.) It was the first time since the formation of the FDA that a drug from the *Cannabis* plant received approval.

LOOKING TO THE FUTURE

In August 2019, the Drug Enforcement Agency (DEA) announced it is "moving forward to facilitate and expand scientific and medical research for marijuana in the United States."[13] To do this, the agency started accepting and reviewing research applications. In September 2019, the U.S. government awarded nine research grants to study CBD in depth. Let's hope research will find CBD helpful for relieving suffering and treating diseases, but only time will tell. It is clearly not the case today.

SUMMARY: AVOID ALL CBD PRODUCTS

Associate Professor of Medicine at Harvard Medical School Dr. Pieter Cohen summarized the advice he gives to his colleagues and his patients in a July 2019 *New England Journal of Medicine* podcast: "Avoid CBD products."[14]

KEY POINTS

Despite a lack of scientific evidence, CBD use is increasing dramatically in the United States due to swelling consumer demand and a steady low-cost supply chain. Although CBD is being promoted for a dizzying number of ailments, it has only been found (in prescription form) to be beneficial in two rare pediatric seizure disorders. Currently, no high-quality studies show benefit in any other disorders.

CBD has known adverse side effects and drug interactions. The short-term and the long-term effects of CBD are largely unknown. Most CBD products are untested and of uncertain purity. Until there are randomized clinical studies showing benefit and standardized regulated products, common sense dictates avoidance of all over-the-counter CBD products.

CITATIONS

1   *https://www.forbes.com/sites/debraborchardt/2016/12/12/the-cannabis-market-that-could-grow-700-by-2020/#4d227a6d4be1*
2   *https://cannabissupplementsforpets.com/*
3   *https://www.christianitytoday.com/ct/2019/may-web-only/some-christians-are-turning-over-new-leaf-with-cbd-oil.html*
4   My local newspaper is the *Daily Progress*, Charlottesville, Virginia
5   Bonn-Miller MO et al., "Labeling Accuracy of Cannabidiol Extracts Sold Online," *JAMA* 2017;318(17):1708-1709.
6   *https://www.pennmedicine.org/news/news-releases/2017/november/penn-study-shows-nearly-70-percent-of-cannabidiol-extracts-sold-online-are-mislabeled*
7   *https://www.forbes.com/sites/janetwburns/2018/05/26/officials-say-fake-cbd-poisoned-at-least-52-people-in-utah-last-winter/#2131236b7dd3*
8   *https://news.vcu.edu/article/Vape_CBD_The_eliquid_might_contain_some_unexpected_ingredients*
9   National Academies of Science, Engineering and Medicine. The Health Effects of Cannabis and Cannabinoids: The Current State of Evidence and Recommendations for Research. Washington, DC: The National Academies Press; 2017.
10 "Cannabidiol for Epilepsy," *The Medical Letter* 2018; 60(1559):182-184.
11 *https://www.fda.gov/news-events/press-announcements/statement-fda-commissioner-scott-gottlieb-md-signing-agriculture-improvement-act-and-agencys*
12 *https://www.cdc.gov/nceh/hsb/success_stories/supplement.htm*
13 *https://www.dea.gov/press-releases/2019/08/26/dea-announces-steps-necessary-improve-access-marijuana-research*
14 *https://www.nejm.org/doi/full/10.1056/NEJMp1906409*

CHAPTER 6

The Current State of
Tetrahydrocannabinol - THC

"That (Marijuana) is not a drug: it's a leaf."
—Arnold Schwarzenegger

Today, despite increasing scientific research suggesting deleterious health issues associated with marijuana, numerous states have legalized recreational and medical marijuana. According to the U.S. National Survey on Drug Use and Health (2018), more than 31 million people have used cannabis in the last month, and more than 53 million people have used marijuana in the last year.[1]

INCREASING USE

Legalization has boosted the number of adult Americans trying THC for the first time, but the increase has not been as great as many had predicted. However, studies show a significant hike among young people and a boost in the frequency of

We haven't legalized marijuana; instead, we have commercialized, capitalized and marketed THC.

use by people who were already users. In 2005, about three million Americans were regular users of THC (more than four times a week); however, that figure has almost tripled today. That means one in every five cannabis users will consume THC daily or almost daily.

IT'S NOT YOUR DAD'S WEED

The levels of THC in marijuana are rising rapidly as industry, eager to meet customer demands for a more rapid and intense high, has created a "new marijuana" rich in THC. One study looked at 38,600 confiscated samples of marijuana taken between the years 1995 and 2014 and found a three-fold rise in THC.[2] While THC concentrations were ballooning from 4% to 12%, CBD levels fell from 0.28% to 0.15%, shifting the THC:CBD ratio from 14X to 80X over those years. Given that CBD tends to mitigate the psychoactive effects of THC, changes in these ratios result in a much more potent substance. THC levels in some plants are now exceeding 30%.[3] That's 10 to 20 times stronger than the marijuana of the 1960s and 1970s. The current marijuana is not your dad's marijuana; in fact, it's a completely different animal.

> THC levels in some plants are now exceeding 30%. That's 10 to 20 times more potent than the marijuana of the 1960s and 1970s. The current marijuana is not your dad's marijuana; in fact, it's a completely different animal.

LET'S DO MORE THAN SMOKE IT

To make matters worse, Americans are now using THC in ways that heighten risks. THC is available in about every form possible (edibles, drinks, suppositories, concentrates, tinctures, creams, etc.) and in strengths that defy imagination. Concentrates, tinctures and oils often contain more than 90% THC producing an intense high when vaporized or dabbed.[4] Consuming THC at these high levels is becoming increasingly common in routine users and presents us with an entirely new set of physical and mental health problems.[5]

In the summer of 2019, thousands of people developed serious lung illnesses from vaping THC. Many were admitted to intensive care units, some required mechanical ventilation (a breathing machine) and some died. The FDA issued a stern warning cautioning people to avoid vaping products with THC oil.

WHAT'S THE BIG DEAL ABOUT HIGHER THC CONCENTRATIONS?

A higher concentration of THC results in a rapid, longer and more vigorous high.

In addition, the psychoactive effects are often different and more dangerous than the effects from a lower dose, which suggests stimulation of additional areas of the brain.

Increased agitation, anxiety, paranoia, psychosis, addiction[6] and other issues are more prevalent with higher THC concentrations.[7] Daily use of high-potency cannabis (defined as THC 10% or greater) was associated with a five-fold increase in the risk for psychosis.[8] Some patients report psychotic episodes long after the last joint. Chronic users of marijuana with high THC content are also at risk for developing the cannabinoid hyperemesis syndrome, which is marked by severe cycles of nausea and vomiting.[9]

With more potent concentrations and frequent use, "desensitization" occurs, which requires users to seek even higher doses in order to achieve the same intensity of high. Even the Netherlands and Uruguay, known for liberal drug laws, are concerned and considering limits on THC concentrations.[10] A bill was introduced in Colorado to limit THC concentrations, but critics of these proposals say the high-potency THC will simply go underground, making it even more dangerous and unregulated.[11]

In states where cannabis is legal, some users prefer extracts, which are nearly pure THC. The comparison between beer and pure grain alcohol pales when we compare marijuana from the 1980s with the extracts of today. To say we have legalized marijuana is misleading; instead, we have commercialized and marketed high potency THC and THC products.

THC and the Young Brain

It is generally accepted that brain development continues until around the age of 25. For instance, the prefrontal cortex doesn't have nearly the functional capacity at age 18 as it does at 25. The studies are clear: the younger a person is when they start using THC, the higher the risk for negative health consequences. This is especially true for physical dependence, addiction, psychosis and the misuse of other substances. The impact on the mental health and educational achievement on our youth cannot be overemphasized in an era where the use of THC by the young is being increasingly normalized.

ADVERSE EFFECTS AND DRUG INTERACTIONS

According to *The Medical Letter* in 2016, adverse effects of THC (dry mouth, sedation, orthostatic hypotension, ataxia and dizziness) occur frequently with medical use of both cannabis and synthetic THC.[12] Anxiety, tachycardia, agitation and confusion are also common, and this can be especially problematic in older patients. THC causes sedation, motor dysfunction, altered perception, cognitive problems and dose-related psychosis. Even low doses of alcohol can significantly raise blood concentrations of THC, thereby intensifying and magnifying all of the side effects. THC is metabolized primarily by CYP2C9 and CYP3A4, and administration with inhibitors of these enzymes may increase the risk of adverse effects.

ADVERSE EFFECTS OF THC ON THOSE UNDER 25 YEARS OF AGE

THC is not a safe drug for those under 25 years of age. The younger the age of exposure to THC, the higher the risk of addiction, mental illness, psychosis, misuse of harder substances, motor vehicle accidents, sexual victimization, academic failure, declines in intelligence measures and occupational impairment. The negative impact of THC on the physical and mental health of our youth cannot be overemphasized in an era where it is being increasingly normalized. (See chapter 24 for additional details.)

DRIVING UNDER THE INFLUENCE OF THC

THC causes impairment in every critical skill set associated with driving a car: coordination, visual tracking, attentiveness, perception of speed, awareness of time, judgment and critical thinking. Because THC is metabolized differently than alcohol, we don't have blood or urine standards or the equivalent of a breath analyzer test to determine a person's level of impairment. To make matters even worse, marijuana-impaired drivers seem to underestimate their level of impairment more than alcohol-impaired drivers, although this is being intensely debated due to conflicting studies. In fact, 70% of marijuana users admit to driving when high, and about the same percentage don't think they will be caught.[13] This confluence of data is disturbing and raises serious public safety issues, especially when we consider the legalization of recreational marijuana.

DECREASED PUBLIC PERCEPTION OF RISK DESPITE INCREASED HOSPITAL EMERGENCY ROOM VISITS

Most Americans today view THC as a safe, medically beneficial chemical being used casually in relaxing social settings. In the 1970s and 80s, when marijuana generally contained less than 5% THC, marijuana users were rarely seen in emergency rooms, but that is no longer the case. Emergency room records from a large hospital in Colorado show a three-fold increase in THC poisonings since the state became the first to allow sales of recreational marijuana.[14] ER visits by people experiencing THC poisoning and overdoses is a daily event in hospitals across the country.

The potency of the "new" marijuana, the upsurge in frequent users and the de-

In the 1970s and 80s, when marijuana generally contained less than 5% THC, marijuana users were rarely seen in emergency rooms for overdoses but that is no longer the case.

creased perception of risk by the public is causing alarm among emergency room personnel, physicians, addiction psychiatrists, psychologists and sociologists around the country for reasons we will explore in upcoming chapters. (See chapters 12, 15, 19 and 20 for additional details.)

FOLLOW THE MONEY: PROFITS OVER PEOPLE

Just like any business selling a product, small businesses, corporations and state governments that profit from sales of THC are looking to boost usage. You can read all the gory details of this massive campaign in Ben Cort's excellent book, *Weed, Inc.*[15] Various advertising and marketing venues—including social media—are skillfully and cunningly used to tout false claims, distort data and increase sales. A recent study examined the website marketing practices of medical and recreational marijuana dispensaries across the U.S., finding that only a few informed the public about risks.[16]

Business schools such as Yale, Wharton and the University of Southern California are devoting faculty and student resources to the emerging marijuana industry. At UCLA, students have even launched the Cannabis Business Association, an official campus club. Sadly, in America, "profits over people" is not an unknown concept or rare practice, even at business schools.

William Wilberforce is generally commended as the person credited with ending slavery throughout the British Empire in the 1800s. Historians have noted that his greatest accomplishment was ending the idea that slavery was an acceptable form of commerce; in other words, he dispelled the notion that slavery was a respectable way to earn a living. For hundreds of years before Wilberforce's time, slavery had been accepted as an economic reality and necessity. Similarly, selling marijuana is rapidly becoming an acceptable way to earn a living in the United States. In many states, keeping or getting marijuana legalized is an economic reality and necessity for small businesses, powerful corporations, investors, various non-profit entities and state governments. This, not unlike the slavery coalitions of old, creates a powerful economic alliance.

Why don't our business schools follow the lead of Wilberforce, demonstrate ethical principles and teach that making a profit from marijuana is not an acceptable form of commerce? Or that selling and promoting THC is not a respectable way to earn a living?

LET'S CALL IT "MEDICINE"

When marijuana advocates and promoters anchored the word "medical" to marijuana without any scientific proof or approval by medical experts, investors saw potential and politicians dreamed of increasing tax revenues. While scientific studies may eventually show health benefits from THC (as is discussed in chapters 5, 6, 7 and 8), that is clearly not the case today.

Some states, like Oklahoma, and Washington D.C. do not even restrict medical marijuana use to specific diseases, which violates the most basic definition of a medication. (Medications are given for a *specific* disorder with *specific* dosing parameters.) When medical marijuana patients decide on their own to "try" cannabis for a particular symptom, true benefit is unlikely, and harm is possible. (See chapter 9 for more details.)

Vulnerable and suffering patients are being misled when they think THC is a medicine. Meanwhile, the profits and tax revenues roll in, making businessmen and politicians happy.

LET'S CALL IT "SOCIAL JUSTICE"

Marijuana advocates have posited legalizing marijuana—selling THC—as a social good. We will discuss this in detail in chapter 17, but let me summarize my opinion succinctly: the poor and disadvantaged will suffer disproportionately just like they have with alcohol, gambling, state-run lotteries and tobacco. The social justice argument is another stratagem by the rich to extract profit from the poor, vulnerable and powerless.

LET'S CALL IT "NATURAL"

Marijuana users like to say how marijuana is "natural" and, therefore, safe and healthy. Although this sounds like a reasonable argument at first glance, the list of things that are natural but dangerous and even deadly could fill an entire chapter. For example, heroin (from the poppy plant), poison ivy (grows in my backyard) and arsenic are all "natural." Enough said. Check out chapter 15 and 22 for additional details.

TWO FDA-APPROVED THC MEDICATIONS

While enthusiasts were espousing implausible arguments that marijuana was medicine, the U.S. government and scientists were quietly funding limited research into possible medicinal uses for THC, and they found two very limited uses: for chemotherapy-induced nausea and for anorexia in patients with wasting diseases. We will discuss nabilone, dronabinol and the FDA approval process in chapter 8.

LOOKING TO THE FUTURE

As noted in the previous chapter on CBD, research and advances in medical science will continue. The Drug Enforcement Agency (DEA) announced it will fund, facilitate and expand scientific and medical research for some of the compounds in marijuana, including THC. Let's hope this research will find THC helpful for relieving more symptoms than the two discussed above.

In the next chapter, we will look at the most recent medical and scientific data and summarize the potential benefits and risks associated with THC.

KEY POINTS

To say we have legalized marijuana is misleading, instead, we have commercialized, capitalized and marketed high potency THC and THC products.

Today, more Americans are using higher potency THC more frequently and in potentially more harmful ways than ever before. The comparison between pure grain alcohol and a beer pales when comparing today's marijuana with the marijuana of the 1970s and 80s.

Despite scientific information to the contrary, most Americans view marijuana as a safe, natural and beneficial medicine. Marijuana advocates—seeking greater profits, personal freedom and tax revenues—have even promoted legalization as a social good, thereby helping consumers feel good about their purchases.

Only recently have the mainstream media and some politicians come to understand the potential risks to individuals and society in our rush to legalize, promote and tax THC products.

CITATIONS

1   Results from the 2018 National Survey on Drug Use and Health: Detailed Tables, SAMHSA, CBHSQ. Accessed on 09/01/19 on *https://www.samhsa.gov/data/sites/default/files/cbhsq-reports/NSDUHDetailedTabs2018R2/NSDUHDetTabsSect1pe2018.htm*

2   ElSohly MA, "Changes in Cannabis Potency Over the Last 2 Decades (1995-2014): Analysis of Current Data in the United States," *Biol Psychiatry* 2016;79(7):613-9.

3   *https://www.cnn.com/2016/10/21/health/colorado-marijuana-potency-above-national-average/index.html*

4   National Institute on Drug Abuse. Marijuana. July 2019. Accessed 9.01.19 at *https://www.drugabuse.gov/marijuana*

5   Monte AA et al., "Acute Illness Associated with Cannabis Use, by Route of Exposure: An Observational Study," *Ann Intern Med* 2019;170(8):531-537.

6   Freeman TP, Winstock AR. Examining the profile of high-potency cannabis and its

association with severity of cannabis dependence. *Psychological Medicine* 2015; 45(15): 3181-9.

7   Volkow ND et al., "Adverse Health Effects of Marijuana Use," *N Engl J Med* 2015;370(23):2219-2227.

8   Di Forti M et al., "The contribution of cannabis use to variation in the incidence of psychotic disorder across Europe: a multicenter case-control study," *Lancet Psychiatry* 2019;6(5):427-436

9   Galli JA et al, "Cannabinoid Hyperemesis Syndrome," *Current Drug Abuse Review* 2011;4(4):241-249.

10   European Monitoring Centre for Drugs and Drug Addiction. Netherlands Country Drug Report 2017. Luxembourg: Publications Office of the European Union; 2017.

11   *https://www.thecannabist.co/2016/03/28/thc-limit-colorado-marijuana/50990/*

12   "Cannabis and Cannabinoids," *The Medical Letter on Drugs and Therapeutics*. August 1, 2016;58(1500):97-98.

13   *https://media.acg.aaa.com/americans-dont-think-theyll-get-arrested-for-driving-high. htm*

14   *https://www.cbsnews.com/news/after-legalization-marijuana-related-er-visits-climb-at-colorado-hospital/*

15   Cort B, *Weed Inc: The Truth about THC, The Pot Lobby and The Commercial Marijuana Industry*, Deerfield Beach, Florida: Healthcare Communications; 2017.

16   Cavazos-Rehg PA, Krauss MJ, Cahn E, et al. Marijuana Promotion Online: an Investigation of Dispensary Practices. *Prev Sci* 2018.

CHAPTER 7

Health Benefits and Risks
Associated with Cannabis

"…conclusive or substantial evidence suggesting that cannabis is effective for the treatment of any medical condition does not presently exist and instead suggests that it may be effective for symptom control only."
—Mayo Clinic Proceedings (2018)[1]

Have you ever heard that marijuana was helpful for glaucoma or dementia or depression? Most Americans have. However, no reasonable studies show any benefit in these conditions;[1] in fact, current evidence shows marijuana being ineffective and possibly harmful in some of these conditions. Maybe you've been told marijuana is helpful in cancer, irritable bowel, epilepsy, Parkinson's and amyotrophic lateral sclerosis (ALS). Actually, there is no reasonable evidence supporting such claims.[2]

On the other hand, it's very possible you heard marijuana causes lung cancer, head and neck cancer, esophageal cancer and asthma. Once again, there is no reasonable evidence for such statements. Perhaps you read marijuana use by parents can cause sudden infant death syndrome, later substance use in their teenage children, leukemia and other tumors in exposed children. There is insufficient or no evidence supporting any of these assertions.[2]

In this chapter, we will explore the health benefits and risks associated with marijuana, but first, let's discuss two important topics: the placebo effect and the significance of anecdotes.

THE PLACEBO EFFECT

The "placebo effect" or "placebo response" is a truly remarkable phenomenon. A fake treatment or inactive substance, like a sugar pill, is given to a person with the expectancy it will help their disease or symptom. Depending on the disposition of the person and the specific disease or symptom being "treated," positive responses—even claims of cure—will occur, ranging from a low of 15% to a high of 72%.

For example, let's say I was to give 100 people a red jellybean and tell them this is a miraculous new drug for helping people sleep longer and deeper. It's virtually guaranteed that the next morning 20% to 30% will say this new drug is truly amazing and they slept like a newborn baby! And, of course, they then tell their family members and friends, and that brings us to our second topic—medical anecdotes.

MEDICAL ANECDOTES

An anecdote is a short interesting story of a real incident or person. In the context of medicine, people will relate with deep emotion and graphic descriptions how some treatment or food or exercise or supplement cured a disease or symptom. Many people find such stories (anecdotes) highly compelling, especially if they suffer with the same ailment. Countless times I've seen well-educated intelligent people do things for health reasons that make absolutely no sense and even cause harm. Physicians and scientists, for extremely good reasons, are deeply suspicious of anecdotal stories; in fact, most of the "miraculous" outcomes are due to the placebo effect. Anecdotes about marijuana's healing prowess are as common as rain in Seattle, Washington.

THE LIMITATIONS OF SCIENCE

In this chapter, we will be looking at the best research available. But it is important to understand that science advances regularly, as new data, novel research and better understanding is the normal progress. What was once considered a weak association by scientists can evolve, because of new studies, into strong evidence, and sometimes what we thought was helpful for a disease actually does harm.

For instance, early studies found that opioid overdose mortality rates between 1999 and 2010 in states allowing medical marijuana use were 21% *lower* than expected.[3] Some concluded that medical marijuana could be an answer to the opioid overdose crisis. When the analysis was extended through 2017, however, they found that the trend reversed, such that states with medical cannabis laws actually experienced an overdose death rate 22.7% *higher* than expected.[4] Indeed, the authors of both studies stated repeatedly that neither study proves evidence of a relationship between marijuana access and opioid overdose deaths; there are simply too many confounding factors. (See chapter 18 for additional details.)

Finally, a number of inherent difficulties are found when gleaning usable information from marijuana research (see sidebar to the right). These include reliability issues, insufficient data and research bias among others. Therefore, future research is needed to provide more definitive answers to questions about the effects of marijuana use.

Marijuana Research

Research on marijuana is hampered by its classification as a Schedule I substance and all of the federal bureaucratic regulations that come with that designation.

Current research on marijuana lacks reliability due to heterogeneity in the active ingredients, the presence of contaminants, poor research methodology, bias, lack of standard dosing, self-reported data and variability in the route of administration.

Definitive studies can only be done with pharmaceutical-grade compounds within randomized controlled trials (RCT).

10,000 STUDIES AND COUNTING

Despite these challenges, numerous short-term and long-term effects of marijuana use are known. In 2017, The National Academies of Sciences, Engineering, and Medicine (NASEM) published a report entitled *The Health Effects of Cannabis and Cannabinoids*. This 468-page document is the most comprehensive and complete literature review ever done and is available online. The committee analyzed more than 10,000 studies and arrived at nearly 100 different research conclusions related to cannabis, cannabinoid use and health.[2]

The committee rated the evidence or association as either substantial, moderate or limited and defined the terms clearly:

Substantial Evidence: There is strong evidence supporting the conclusion or association. For this level of evidence, there must be several good quality studies with few or no credible opposing findings.

Moderate Evidence: There is some evidence supporting the conclusion or association. For this level of evidence, there must be several good-to-fair studies with few or no credible opposing findings.

Limited Evidence: There is weak evidence supporting the conclusion or association. For this level of evidence, there must be several fair quality studies or mixed findings with most favoring the conclusion or association.

For Those Under 25 Years of Age

The research is unequivocal: the younger the age of initiation to marijuana, the higher the risk of all of the negative health consequences described in this chapter. This is worrisome in a culture where teen and college age use of marijuana is being increasingly normalized.

In this chapter, I have decided to only list NASEM conclusions that can be backed by substantial or moderate evidence. At this point, it is important to mention there is a battle for public perception. Sadly, people on both sides are distorting and manipulating research results, and this is generally done by over-emphasizing weak, biased or small studies or by touting anecdotal stories as proof. Therefore, I will not be listing any studies with limited or weak evidence in this chapter.

It is worth noting that marijuana has not cured or effectively treated a single medical condition. When it helps, it only reduces the symptoms. In a December 2018 article in *Mayo Clinic Proceedings*, the authors said, "conclusive or substantial evidence suggesting that cannabis is effective for the treatment of any medical condition does not presently exist and instead suggests that it may be effective for symptom control only."[1]

POSITIVE HEALTH OUTCOMES AND THERAPEUTIC EFFECTS ASSOCIATED WITH CANNABIS[2]

Substantial (Strong) Evidence For:
- *Treating chemotherapy-induced nausea and vomiting (oral prescription medications)*
- *Treating chronic pain in adults (cannabis)*
- *Improving patient-reported spasticity in multiple sclerosis*

There is substantial evidence for the oral treatment of chemotherapy-induced nausea and vomiting. As previously mentioned, two FDA-approved oral medications are derived from marijuana—dronabinol and nabilone—specifically for these two conditions (see chapter 8). No evidence supports self-medication for nausea or vomiting with marijuana.

There is substantial evidence that marijuana is effective in the treatment of chronic pain, but the FDA has not approved it for this indication. More than 20 studies have been done on chronic and neuropathic pain, with positive results in about half of them. Randomized trials of cannabinoids have found some evidence of efficacy for second-line treatment of cancer and neuropathic pain. A fairly large study of more than 1,500 patients found that cannabis did not improve outcomes or reduce prescription opioid use in patients with chronic non-cancer pain.[5] No good head-to-head studies compare cannabis with other pain relief drugs like ibuprofen.

Substantial evidence shows that marijuana is effective in the treatment of patient-reported spasticity in multiple sclerosis, but the FDA has not approved it for this condition. More than 30 studies have been completed with multiple sclerosis, and cannabis was found to only be helpful where patients were asked to monitor and report changes in the spasticity themselves. Third-party observers did not see improvement. There was not enough evidence to recommend cannabis or cannabinoids for spasticity in patients with spinal cord injury. Skeptics have pointed out that most hallucinogenic and sedative medications (alcohol, benzodiazepines, opioids, etc.) will reduce patient-reported spasms.

Moderate (Some) Evidence For:
- *Improving sleep outcomes in patients with obstructive sleep apnea syndrome, fibromyalgia, chronic pain and multiple sclerosis*
- *Improving cognitive performance among individuals with psychotic disorders who also had a previous history of cannabis use*

Improvements in sleep were seen mainly in studies with oral nabiximols (Sativex), a prescription combination product not yet available in the United States (see chapter 8 for more details on Sativex.)

Finally, some evidence shows marijuana improved cognitive performance among individuals with psychotic disorders who also had a previous history of cannabis use. Clearly, this is a complex area. Most medical journals, like the *Mayo Clinic Proceedings*,[1] do not even list this as a positive therapeutic effect. Obviously, any therapeutic actions taken because of this finding should be initiated by addiction psychiatrists only.

NEGATIVE HEALTH OUTCOMES ASSOCIATED WITH CANNABIS[2]

Substantial (Strong) Evidence For:
- *More frequent and more severe episodes of chronic bronchitis (long-term cannabis smoking)*
- *Increased risk of motor vehicle accidents*
- *Low birth weight in newborns (maternal smoking)*
- *Development of schizophrenia and other psychoses*

Moderate (Some) Evidence For:

- *Impairment in the cognitive domains of learning, memory and attention (acute cannabis use)*
- *Increased incidence of suicidal ideation and suicide attempts (higher incidence among heavy users)*
- *Increased incidence of suicide completion*
- *Increased incidence of social anxiety disorder (regular cannabis use)*
- *Worsening of bipolar symptoms (regular cannabis use)*
- *Pediatric overdose injuries*
- *Small increased risk for depression*
- *Increased severity of post-traumatic stress disorder symptoms (problem cannabis use)*
- *Development of a substance use disorder for other substances (alcohol, nicotine and other illicit drugs)*

We will be discussing the harmful effects of marijuana in more detail in chapter 15.

TAKEAWAYS FROM THE NASEM STUDIES, SELF-TREATMENT AND FALSE HOPES

It's very possible your state's medical marijuana laws specifically approve medical marijuana as treatment for illnesses such as HIV, ALS, hepatitis, Parkinson's, cancer and glaucoma, even though the data from scientific studies was weak, nonexistent or even suggested harm.[1] For instance, most states include ALS on their list of approved illnesses for medical marijuana, despite the fact that there have been only two small randomized double-blind clinical studies and the results of effectiveness were unequivocally negative and showed there was no benefit.

The sad truth is that approved diagnoses for medical marijuana are not based on reputable studies and reports like NASEM. Instead, they were written by professional lobbyists and well-paid attorneys who were seemingly oblivious to the fact they would be exposing millions to fraudulent advertising, false hopes and risky self-treatment (see chapter 9 for more information).

In his book *Weed, Inc.*, Ben Cort tells the story of a man who had a serious brain tumor and wanted to smoke marijuana to help cure his tumor.[6] Evidently, he read a report that showed synthesized CBD, at about 10,000 times the potency found in a plant, reduced the size and growth of some brain tumors. The message he heard was, "Marijuana cures brain tumors," which is a far cry from the reality of that study. Unfortunately, some states have even included gliomas (a type of brain tumor) on their approved list for medical marijuana despite zero evidence (see chapters 9 and 15).

Some experts have criticized the NASEM studies for not emphasizing the added risks marijuana poses to those under 25 years of age. Research and science have revealed that teens and young people are neurologically, psychologically and socially different than adults. Their brains are still developing and, consequently, cannabis poses a much greater risk to young people than adults.

KEY POINTS

There are symptom-relief benefits and genuine risks from the chemicals contained in the *Cannabis* plant, which are outlined in this chapter. However, politics, policy and accessibility have leaped far ahead of medical science, thereby exposing millions to fraudulent health claims and dangerous self-treatment.

There is no conclusive evidence currently that cannabis is effective for the cure of any medical condition; however, it may be effective for symptom control in some extremely limited conditions.

Additional research conducted with pharmaceutical-grade marijuana-derived substances is the best path forward to finding more positive health benefits and understanding the true risks of this intriguing plant. People should exercise caution by carefully considering the risks and benefits when considering marijuana use.

CITATIONS

1   Ebbert J et al., "Medical Cannabis," *Mayo Clinic Proceedings* 2018; 93(12):1842-1847.
2   National Academies of Science, Engineering and Medicine. The Health Effects of Cannabis and Cannabinoids: The Current State of Evidence and Recommendations for Research. Washington, DC: The National Academies Press; 2017.
3   Bachhuber M et al., "Medical Cannabis Laws and Opioid Analgesic Overdose Mortality in the United States, 1999–2010," *JAMA Intern Med* 2014; 174(10): 1668–1673.
4   Shover at al., "Association between medical cannabis laws and opioid overdose mortality has reversed over time" *Proceedings of the National Academy of Science* 2019; 116(26): 12624-12626.
5   Campbell G et al., "Effect of cannabis use in people with chronic non-cancer pain prescribed opioids: findings from a 4-year prospective cohort study," *Lancet Public Health* 2018; 3(7): 341-350.
6   Cort B, *Weed Inc: The truth about the THC, the pot lobby, and the commercial marijuana industry*. Deerfield Beach, Florida: Health Communications; 2017.

Politics, Policies and Precepts

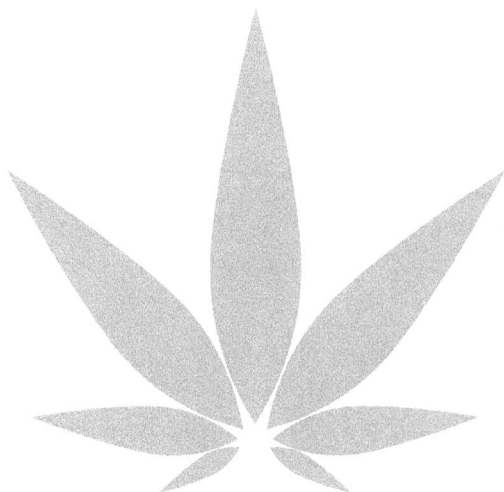

"The only lesson you can learn from
history is that it repeats itself."
—Bangambiki Habyarimana, *The Great Pearl of Wisdom*

SECTION 3

POLITICS, POLICIES AND PRECEPTS

Foxglove is a beautiful garden plant, and it surrounds my mailbox. *Digitalis*, the genus name, describes the finger-like appearance of its flowers. The pinkish-purplish bells, spotted throats and graceful stems cheer my wife and me up every time we pick up the mail. Foxglove also gives us the perfect story to introduce the concept of marijuana as medicine.

Foxglove was considered a toxic plant for centuries because people and animals who ate the plant tended to have vomiting, nausea, dizziness, hallucinations, abdominal pain and diarrhea. Some even died. Myths arose and some people referred to the plant as "witch's glove," emphatically warning every one of its potential toxicity. Positive health anecdotes, however, persisted and foxglove eventually found its way into folk medicine in the 1600s. It was recommended for a host of diseases and symptoms, but reports of deaths, increased sickness and cures were confounding and perplexing.

In the mid-1700s, British physician William Withering studied the plant after hearing about an "old woman in Shropshire" who insisted that eating the plant improved her health. Convinced of its benefits after doing research, Withering published in 1785 a book entitled *An Account of the Foxglove and Some of Its Medical Uses: With Practical Remarks on Dropsy, and Other Diseases*. He believed correctly that the *Digitalis* plant was good for "dropsy," which is known today as "heart failure."

His book sparked a renewed interest in foxglove as a possible medicinal candidate. From the 1800s through the mid-1900s, researchers isolated the active ingredient (digoxin), purified it, tested it and found it strengthened the contractions of the heart muscle and slowed down the heart rate. Researchers and physicians tested absorption and determined the correct dose for humans for each indication. The amount needed for atrial fibrillation tended to be higher than the amount needed for heart failure. Specialists in manufacturing then developed the processes needed for precise dosing. It was quickly designated as a prescription-only medicine, meaning a physician had to give permission before a patient could use it. Prescription medications, because they are either powerful or dangerous, are not available over the counter or licensed for sale to the general public. They go through a rigorous approval process (which we will describe in the next chapter), require a physician's prescription and must be dispensed by a licensed pharmacist.

As a prescription medication, digoxin went on to relieve the suffering of millions of patients with heart failure and atrial fibrillation. However, new obstacles soon developed. Digoxin needed to be taken frequently to be effective, and physicians found that toxic quantities were only a bit higher than therapeutic doses. Blood tests were then developed to monitor the blood levels so doses could be adjusted precisely, while long-acting compounds were developed to make compliance easier. Because of these improvements, digoxin is still prescribed today.

But what if we had kept on growing foxglove in our backyards? What if everyone experimented by themselves and tried to figure out what to use it for, when to use it, how often to use it and how much to use?

One of the things we will be referring to with regard to medical marijuana is the shortage of good medical studies, little to no dose standardization and an almost complete absence of knowledge as to what diseases and conditions it might benefit. Despite this, numerous states have passed laws allowing medical marijuana for a wide host of diseases, while some states say it can be recommended for any and all conditions. Although the analogy isn't perfect, today's situation with marijuana almost sounds like foxglove in the 1600s.

As hundreds of years of research and experience have shown, digitalis ultimately had a very limited role to play in medicine. It was only helpful in heart failure and atrial fibrillation. The dosing had to be precise. In fact, when not carefully monitored, digoxin often hurt other organs like the kidneys, brain and gastrointestinal system. In states that have passed medical marijuana laws, we are giving a poorly understood herb to large numbers of people as "medicine" *before* research and physicians have established the indications, safety, dosing, frequency and effectiveness. We are subjecting thousands and thousands of people to fraudulent health claims and unsafe self-medication practices. This is not how medicine is supposed to function. In the next four chapters, let's look at four public policy approaches to marijuana: FDA-approved marijuana medications, state-sanctioned medical marijuana, recreational marijuana and the decriminalization of marijuana.

CHAPTER 8

FDA-Approved Marijuana Medications

"At the FDA, our mission is to promote and protect the health of the public. As commissioner, I've worked hard to galvanize people around that idea. I want employees to be thinking about the unique and essential contribution they are making to our mission."
—Margaret Ann Hamburg, MD,
Chair of the Board of the American Association for the Advancement of Science and the 21st Commissioner of the U.S. Food and Drug Administration

It is not widely known that there are three cannabinoid medications available by prescription in the United States: nabilone (Cesamet), dronabinol (Marinol and Syndros) and cannabidiol (Epidiolex). These medications are pharmaceutical-grade and quality-controlled, and they are dosed and indicated for specific conditions and diagnoses.

WHY DO WE NEED FDA-APPROVED PRESCRIPTION CANNABINOID DRUGS?

Why would a person take a cannabinoid drug when they can simply use marijuana? If you think back to chapter 2, the marijuana plant contains numerous types of cannabinoids as well as other compounds, including pesticides and contaminants. Some of these may be harmful and cause undesired side effects. So, when scientists believe they have found a plant that can help people, they try to identify the useful substances in the plant, isolate them, learn to manufacture them and improve them. Many of our current medications have been found this way like digoxin (from foxglove).

Similar to digoxin, the three cannabinoid drugs we are going to discuss in this chapter have been carefully isolated, purified, manufactured, dosed and tested. If we don't get the dose right at first (after all, every individual is different), we can adjust and control it readily, knowing precisely the milligram dose we are giving. In a naturally diverse and heterogenous product like a plant, the dose or strength may vary significantly.

FDA APPROVAL: AN ARDUOUS PROCESS

Before these three prescription medications were released to the public, they had to get approval from the Food and Drug Administration (FDA), the federal agency charged with approving the production and sale of prescription medications. Getting a drug approved is not for the faint of heart; in fact, it's an arduous process (see sidebar on next page).[1]

All three of these medications endured extensive animal research, and when they went well, clinical trials in humans followed. These medications were then accurately dosed for specific conditions and diagnoses—down to the milligram. Maximum doses were established. Drug interactions were studied. Public hearings were held. After all of this was accomplished, the FDA considered them for approval and assigned a Controlled Substances Schedule Level (see the chart at the end of this chapter). Even today, these medications are closely regulated from the chemistry lab to the pharmacy. Testing and re-evaluations will continue indefinitely to ensure these prescription medications remain safe and efficacious. In fact, much of what we know about THC and CBD is due to this proven process.

1. **Nabilone (Cesamet)** is a synthetic THC medication that received FDA approval in 1985 for the treatment of chemotherapy-induced nausea and vomiting that has not responded to other antiemetic treatments. Nabilone is Schedule II under the Controlled Substances Act and is therefore considered to have a high potential for abuse.

2. **Dronabinol (Marinol, Syndros and generics)** is another synthetic THC medication, and it received FDA approval seven years after nabilone in 1992 for (1) the treatment of chemotherapy-induced nausea and vomiting that has not responded to other antiemetic treatments; and (2) to treat anorexia in patients with wasting diseases, such as AIDS. Dronabinol is Schedule III under the Controlled Substances Act, as individuals receiving the drug for treatment have reported both psychological and physiological dependence.

In neither of these indications is nabilone or dronabinol considered the best or first-line medication. For example, for patients experiencing severe nausea from severely emetogenic (nausea-causing) chemotherapy drugs, the FDA-approved drugs palonosetron (Aloxi) and aprepitant (Emend) are more effective and better tolerated than dronabinol and nabilone.

3. **Cannabidiol (Epidiolex):** In June 2018, the FDA approved the first natural marijuana plant-derived drug, Epidiolex. It only contains CBD—no THC. It is available by prescription as an oil for the treatment of seizures associated with two rare forms of childhood epilepsy: Lennox-Gastaut Syndrome (LGS) and Dravet Syndrome. Current research does not support or recommend cannabidiol for the treatment of patients with more common types of epilepsy. Epidiolex has been approved as a Schedule V controlled substance by the DEA. (Schedule V substances are the least restrictive schedule of the controlled substances.)

When you pick up one of these medications from the pharmacy, you will leave the pharmacy well-informed. You will know what dose to take (to the precise milligram), what symptoms or diseases it treats, a list of potential side effects, food or drug interactions and an expiration date. You will take the medication with peace of mind knowing the medication is carefully regulated and monitored. As we will see in the next chapter, this is not the case with medical marijuana.

OFF-LABEL USE

Currently, there are no other FDA-approved uses for the marijuana plant. However, physicians may prescribe any of these for other conditions and diagnoses. This is called "prescribing a medication off-label use." The off-label use of medications is common in the U.S., and up to one-fifth of prescriptions are prescribed off-label. Among psychiatric drugs, off-label prescribing is about 30%.[2]

The ability to prescribe drugs for uses beyond the officially approved conditions is used by physicians for the patient's benefit. This enables physicians to give a medication for an unapproved condition while the manufacturer completes or contemplates new clinical trials.

As might be expected, off-label use can entail increased health risks to the patient and increased legal liability for the physician. Research suggests that off-label prescribing may have a higher incidence of adverse side effects. Consequently, most physicians will only prescribe a medication "off-label" when they are convinced it is safe, efficacious and an accepted medical practice.

THE FUTURE

Currently, pharmaceutical companies are doing additional research and working to gain FDA approval for marijuana-derived medications for use in multiple sclerosis and pain. One of these, nabiximols (Sativex) seems promising. It is a 1:1 THC/

Steps to Prescription FDA Medication Approval

Preclinical Studies: Theories about possible benefits and side effects from a drug are formulated and followed by laboratory studies in animals. Safety and efficacy are carefully evaluated before proceeding to human trials.

Phase 1 Trials are meant to evaluate the safety of the new drug in humans. The first patients in a Phase 1 Trial are assigned a dose that is a fraction of what could safely be given to animals; in fact, these small doses are unlikely to benefit a patient. Doses are slowly increased while researchers evaluate the absorption, metabolism and excretion of the drug. Researchers carefully document all side effects.

Phase 2 Trials evaluate whether a new drug works as postulated in the animal studies. Safety is still monitored, but therapeutic value is now the primary endpoint. These researchers are looking for even small signs of benefit as most patients on Phase 2 Trials have typically failed standard treatments. When Phase 2 Trials end, investigators will look at their results and decide whether they will proceed to the larger and more expensive Phase 3 Trials. Many companies will abandon the drug after Phase 2 if the results are not convincing.

Phase 3 Trials are much more costly as they need to include enough patients to determine if a new drug is better than the standard treatment. The gold standard for a Phase 3 Trial is the randomized control trial, which we explained in a sidebar in chapter 5. The FDA makes decisions on approval of a drug after the completion of one or more Phase 3 Trials.

Phase 4 Trials: Sometimes after analyzing the data from the first three phases of clinical trials, the FDA will approve a drug but ask for a Phase 4 Trial. This is sometimes referred to as a post-marketing study because it is used to learn more about a drug after it has been approved and publicly available. Phase 4 Trials allow the investigators to follow any adverse effects.

CBD mixture and is already available by prescription in Canada, Australia, the United Kingdom and Spain.[3]

Scientists are also conducting preclinical and clinical trials with marijuana and its extracts to treat symptoms of illness and other conditions, such as HIV/AIDS, cancer, multiple sclerosis (MS), inflammation, pain, seizures, substance use disorders and mental disorders.[4]

Some basic science researchers, including those funded by the National Institutes of Health (NIH), are exploring the possible uses of THC, CBD and other cannabinoids for numerous other conditions.

RECOMMENDATIONS

Because cannabis is classified as a Schedule I drug under federal law, research has been hampered. Unfortunately, this lack of information hasn't stopped patients from exploring the use of cannabis on their own. Ideally, in the future the FDA should consider rescheduling marijuana to a Schedule II drug (the same category as cocaine and fentanyl) to facilitate and accelerate research and knowledge.

CONTROLLED SUBSTANCES ACT SCHEDULING

Schedule	Description of Substances	Examples
I	No accepted medical use and a high potential for abuse	Heroin, LSD, marijuana
II	High potential for abuse with risk of severe psychological or physical dependence	Vicodin, hydromorphone, meperidine, cocaine, fentanyl, Ritalin
III	Moderate to low potential for physical and psychological dependence. Abuse potential less than Schedule I and Schedule II, but more than IV.	Products with < 90 mg codeine per dose (Tylenol with codeine), ketamine, anabolic steroids
IV	Low potentials for abuse and risk of dependence	Xanax, Soma, Darvon, Valium, Ativan, Ambien, Tramadol
V	Lower potential for abuse than Schedule IV; preparations containing limited quantities of certain narcotics. Generally used for antidiarrheal, antitussive and analgesic purposes.	Cough preparations with < 200 mg codeine or per 100 mL (Robitussin AC), Lomotil, Motofen, Lyrica, Parepectolin

Adapted from DEA. Drug Scheduling. *https://www.dea.gov/drug-scheduling* (accessed February 7, 2019).

KEY POINTS

There are three FDA-approved cannabinoid medications, and all are dosed and indicated for specific conditions and diagnoses. These medications are pharmaceutical-grade THC or CBD, are manufactured to precise milligram amounts, are guaranteed to not contain any contaminants or other compounds and are closely regulated from production to distribution.

These three medications demonstrate the best way to legalize marijuana products intended for use as medicine. Rather than legalizing a medicine by popular vote and political lobbying (as is being done with medical marijuana currently), we should limit the uses of marijuana for medicine through the FDA-approval process described above. Formal clinical studies and randomized controlled trials can definitely demonstrate medical efficacy and safety, potentially benefiting millions of people in the future.

CITATIONS

1   *https://www.fda.gov/drugs/development-approval-process-drugs*
2   Radley DC et al., "Off-label Prescribing Among Office-Based Physicians," *Archives of Internal Medicine* 2006;166 (9): 1021–1026.
3   *https://www.gwpharm.com/healthcare-professionals/sativex*
4   National Institute on Drug Abuse. Marijuana. July 2019. Accessed 9.01.19 at *https://www.drugabuse.gov/marijuana.*

CHAPTER 9

The Legalization of Medical Marijuana

"I want you to hear me say this as the nation's doctor:
there is no such thing as medical marijuana."
—Surgeon General of the United States Jerome Adams, MD (June 2019)

"There is no such thing as medical marijuana."
—U.S. Health and Human Services Secretary Alex Azar (March 2018)

Medical marijuana is the use of the leaves, flowers, buds or extracts of the *Cannabis* plant to treat diseases or symptoms. As of October 2019, 33 states (plus the District of Columbia, Guam, Puerto Rico and the U.S. Virgin Islands) have legalized medical marijuana, although the United States Federal Government still classifies marijuana as a Schedule I drug with no current accepted medical use.

DRUG SCHEDULES

In 1970, the U.S. Congress passed the Controlled Substances Act (CSA). The CSA drug scheduling system forms the backbone of our government's drug policy as it places all drugs—legal and illegal—into the five classifications we referenced earlier: Schedule I to Schedule V.

Since the early 1970s, marijuana has been classified as a Schedule I drug, which puts it in the most circumscribed category along with drugs like heroin and LSD.

Surprisingly to some, cocaine and methamphetamine are in Schedule II, a less restrictive category. But that doesn't mean the federal government views marijuana as more dangerous than meth or cocaine. The key difference between Schedule I and II substances is whether a drug has medicinal value or not. Schedule II substances are deemed to have some medicinal value, while Schedule I drugs do not; therefore, the government puts tighter restrictions on those classified as Schedule I.

Think of the scheduling system as being divided into two distinct groups: "non-medical" and "medical." The "non-medical group" is the Schedule I drugs, as they have no medicinal value and a high potential for abuse. The "medical group" is the Schedule II to V drugs, as they have some medicinal value and are numerically ranked based on abuse potential. Schedule II drugs have a high potential for abuse (for example, opioids are in Schedule II) and Schedule V drugs have a low potential for abuse (for example, antidiarrheal medications are Schedule V).

The division between "non-medical" and "medical" is not academic. **The fundamental issue of this entire chapter rests on this question: should marijuana be considered a legitimate medicine or not?**

MEDICAL MARIJUANA BASICS

In order to purchase marijuana for medical purposes, a person must go to a state-licensed medical marijuana dispensary (not a pharmacy), prove residency in that state, demonstrate that he or she meets the minimum age (typically 18 or 21, depending on the state), pass a brief background check (in some states) and present a physician certification. A physician certification is a form filled out by a physician to "certify" a patient for one of the approved medical marijuana conditions. (The physician is not providing a prescription, as he or she is simply attesting that a certain condition exists.)

A CHANGE IN STRATEGY: "FREEDOM AND AUTONOMY" TO "BENEFICIAL MEDICINE"

As we discussed in previous chapters, when marijuana proponents anchored the word "medical" to marijuana, there was a boost in public acceptance and, despite opposition from the medical and scientific communities, medical marijuana became common parlance.

But not for everyone. Attaching the word "medical" to marijuana triggered confusion among patients, nurses, the public and even physicians as "medical marijuana" became muddled with the FDA-approved marijuana-derived medications we discussed in chapter 8.

The United States Food and Drug Administration's (FDA) process for approving and regulating drugs is the envy of the world, as American medications are widely recognized for their precise standardization, production, packaging, distribution

> "There's a certain libertarian...view that there should be no FDA, that people can decide for themselves whether medicines are safe and effective. That's nonsense. Most people don't have the expertise or the resources to mount a proper study to find out whether a treatment is safe or effective."
> —Marcia Angell, MD, American physician and the first woman to serve as editor-in-chief of the *New England Journal of Medicine*[2]

and safety. On the other hand, because it is not legal by federal law, medical marijuana is not regulated by the FDA. Instead, management and administration are left to the individual states.

Lacking the resources and know how, state legalization of medical marijuana has not been accompanied by the rigorous scientific approval process that has made FDA-approved medications respected. In almost all states, medical marijuana has been approved for conditions[1] where research is inadequate.[2] Therefore, the safety and efficacy of medical marijuana is illusory.

Unknowing patients, assuming that state dispensaries are tightly monitored like pharmacies, are not aware that using medical marijuana can result in addiction, psychosis, mental or psychosocial impairment, lung damage and heart attacks, to name just a few (see chapters 7, 15, 16, 19, 20, 23 and 24).

THERE IS NO SUCH THING AS MEDICAL MARIJUANA

As we have discussed in preceding chapters, the science supporting the concept of medical marijuana is deficient. On March 2, 2018, U.S. Health and Human Services Secretary Alex Azar said, "There really is no such thing as medical marijuana."[3] On June 24, 2019, Surgeon General of the United States Dr. Jerome Adams stated emphatically, "I want you to hear me say this as the nation's doctor: there is no such thing as medical marijuana."[4]

The FDA does not recognize, regulate or approve the marijuana plant as medicine. "Researchers haven't conducted enough large-scale clinical trials that show that the

> "We at the Cleveland Clinic...will not be recommending 'medical marijuana' for our patients...we believe there are better alternatives."
> —Paul Terpeluk, DO, Medical Director of Cleveland Clinic's Employee Health Services[6]

benefits of the marijuana plant outweigh its risks in patients it's meant to treat," as written by the National Institute on Drug Abuse.[5]

The Cleveland Clinic, Johns Hopkins and other reputable hospitals have spoken out against medical marijuana. Medical Director at the Cleveland Clinic Dr. Paul Terpeluk summarized their position this way in January 2019: "In the world of healthcare, a medication is a drug that has endured extensive clinical trials, public hearings and approval by the U.S. Food & Drug Administration (FDA). Medications are tested for safety and efficacy. They are closely regulated, from production to distribution. They are accurately dosed, down to the milligram. Medical marijuana is none of those things."[6]

On August 29, 2019, Surgeon General Adams issued a rare public warning about marijuana, stressing the public's lack of awareness, its effects on the brain and the dramatic increase in marijuana's potency. He also emphasized the risk of marijuana to teens and the unborn child.[7]

QUESTIONABLE APPROVED DIAGNOSES AND INDICATIONS

Several states have approved marijuana as treatment for illnesses such as HIV, ALS, hepatitis, Parkinson's, Alzheimer's, cancer and glaucoma, even though the data from scientific studies is weak, nonexistent or demonstrates harm for these same diseases.[8]

As we have mentioned before, the state-approved diagnoses for marijuana use were not written by physicians or experts in the field; instead, they were written by professional lobbyists and hired lawyers.[9]

Finally, the Cleveland Clinic stated in its medical marijuana statement that "there are better alternatives" for every listed condition and symptom in the state medical marijuana laws.[6]

Some physicians are even acting negligently. A study in the *Journal of Clinical Oncology* in 2018 found that almost one-half of cancer doctors admitted recommending medical marijuana to their patients, although most confessed they lacked the necessary evidence to do so.[10] This study was especially disturbing given that no major medical association has even endorsed the concept that marijuana can be a medicine.

Physicians cannot assume that medical marijuana is safe or effective for state-listed qualifying diseases or conditions, nor can they be sure it contains the labeled amount of active ingredient. They can't even be sure it is devoid of contaminants, pesticides and harmful additives. Kleber and DuPont summarized the situation well in a 2012 commentary in the *American Journal of Psychiatry*: "Medical marijuana laws challenge physicians to recommend use of a Schedule 1 illegal drug of abuse with no scientific approval, dosage control, or quality control."[11]

POLITICS, PROFITS AND POPULARITY TRUMP MEDI-CINE AND SCIENCE

Never before has an herb been legalized as "medicine" by popular vote. Politics, profits, celebrity popularity and personal freedom claims have trumped rational thought, science and medicine.[12]

On September 8, 2019, the *Washington Post* posted an analysis of Maryland's medical marijuana program: "Industry analysts had predicted the market would gross $60 million in sales by its third year. But by the end of its first year, in December, purveyors' gross sales surpassed $96 million. Then lawmakers authorized the sale of edible cannabis products…Regulators noted that there is still substantial room for growth in the medical cannabis market in Maryland, which has opened 82 dispensaries across the state in less than two years."[13] This is not a few hippie farmers or health enthusiasts growing marijuana. This is big business. Notice how the state grades its operations on sales. In other words, the state of Maryland is hoping for more users so it can claim success by reporting increased tax revenues. "Tax revenues are more important than the health of our people" seems to be the priority of state officials as perverse incentives abound.

"IF WEED IS MEDICINE, SO IS BUDWEISER"

Dr. Bach of Memorial Sloan-Kettering, entitled his op-ed piece in the *Wall Street Journal*, "If Weed is Medicine, So is Budweiser" to make a point.[14] For instance, what was the main ingredient in all medications before the modern age of medicine? (Think about peddlers selling snake oil.) Alcohol. It reduced pain, helped headaches, relieved muscle aches, helped people relax, improved sleep, etc., but do we consider alcohol a medicine today? Of course not. Dr. Bach and others believe some of the substances in the marijuana plant may have medicinal benefits, but the marijuana plant as a whole should not be considered a medicine. It is more akin to alcohol than medicine.

INCREASED COMMUNITY ACCESS AND A SLIPPERY SLOPE TO RECREATIONAL MARIJUANA

Evidence suggests that the increase in availability and accessibility in states where medical marijuana is legal is leading to an increase in recreational usage.[15] States with legal medical marijuana have youth usage rates surpassing those in states that do not. One study from Oregon found that communities with a greater number of medical marijuana patients were associated with a higher prevalence of marijuana use among youth. The authors speculated that more accepting community attitudes in these areas could be influencing teen behaviors. Other studies have noted equivocal or contrasting findings.[16,17]

The Number of Marijuana Users in a State Decreases as We Go Down This List:

- Recreational marijuana is legal
- Medical marijuana is legal
- Marijuana is decriminalized
- Marijuana classified as illegal

The approval of medical marijuana has been a stepping stone to approving recreational marijuana. Every single state that has legalized recreational marijuana actually legalized medical marijuana first.

"SMOKING A MEDICATION" IS AN OXYMORON

Smoking is a harmful route of administration for any medicinal compound because of carcinogens and other harmful materials which are known to produce adverse effects on the lungs and other tissues.[2,18,19,20] No prudent or reasonable physician or healthcare professional should ever recommend smoking as an accepted delivery vehicle for a medicine. Period.

MY POSITION ON LEGALIZING MEDICAL MARIJUANA

In my opinion, marijuana is not a legitimate medicine. Medical marijuana is an oxymoron, like "open secret" or "lead balloon."

I oppose the legalization of medical marijuana for the following reasons:

1. There are inadequate research and clinical trials.
2. Studies show questionable efficacy.
3. There are better alternatives for every symptom or disease.
4. FDA-approved medications (see chapter 8) derived from marijuana are superior.
5. Production, distribution and dosing are not regulated or standardized.
6. There is no short-term or long-term safety record.
7. Smoking any medication for health is a self-contradiction as all smoking is unhealthy.
8. It creates a false perception of marijuana as a beneficial substance.
9. It subjects people to fraudulent health claims.
10. It encourages potentially dangerous self-treatment of genuine diseases.
11. It increases access to marijuana use in the community, including vulnerable populations.
12. It creates a legislative stepping stone to recreational marijuana.

MY RECOMMENDATIONS

1. Vote "No" on medical marijuana referendums.
2. Reschedule marijuana to Schedule II to accelerate research and allow FDA and federal involvement in regulating marijuana.
3. Encourage the development of marijuana-derived medicine via the standard FDA approval process for all medications.
4. Recognize that medical conditions are best treated with FDA-approved medications.
5. If you live in a state where medical marijuana is legal, encourage the rewriting of medical marijuana laws to:
    a. Limit THC to under 15%.
    b. Protect consumers from false advertising and self-treatment.
    c. Develop programs to prevent driving while intoxicated.
    d. Develop strategies to prevent access to teens, young people and pregnant moms.
    e. Crack down on those accessing medical marijuana for the purpose of selling it in the community.
    f. Establish harsh penalties for those selling cannabis to minors.
    g. Continue aggressive measures against those growing, distributing and selling marijuana illegally.
    h. Increase education of the public.
6. Refrain from using medical marijuana yourself, even if it is legalized, and take a vocal position against the legalization of medical marijuana.

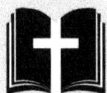

THE CHRISTIAN PERSPECTIVE
MARIJUANA AS MEDICINE

A Christian perspective for using marijuana as a medicine requires a summary of four principles: (1) medicine as a potential good; (2) submission to government and authorities; (3) praying for government leaders; and (4) a higher standard for Christian physicians.

MEDICINE AS A POTENTIAL GOOD

Scripture seems to encourage prayer, anointing with oil, common sense and medical treatment for ailments. In Proverbs 31 and 1 Timothy, we see King Lemuel and Paul recommending common sense and medicine for the sole purpose of ameliorating physical ailments. Luke, one of the writers of the fourth Gospel, was a physician. Jesus clearly viewed physical healing as a good, and He demonstrated this emphatically by healing on the Sabbath. From these and other verses, medical treatment seems to be viewed in the Bible as an extension of God's mercy to those who are suffering or hurting. In other words, Christians may seek and experience the Lord's healing hand through the help of knowledgeable and trained physicians. Finally, and expectantly, believers look forward to that glorious day when all death, crying and suffering is destroyed, and medicine will no longer be needed.

SUBMISSION TO GOVERNMENTS AND AUTHORITIES

Scripture calls Christians to be submissive to governments and authorities (Romans 13:2-7; 1 Peter 2:17-18). Since no government or authority is perfect or flawless, there clearly are limits to this submissiveness when the authorities and biblical commands are in conflict. In the case of medical marijuana, the mandate is clear: Christians living in jurisdictions forbidding marijuana use should obey those laws. The rest of this book is addressed to those living in jurisdictions where medical marijuana is legal, because they need to delve deeper into the issues.

PRAYING FOR GOVERNMENT LEADERS

We are called to pray for our leaders. We are serving God by honoring the system of government He established by praying for those in authority over us (Romans 13:1; 1 Timothy 2:1-2). Before writing this book, I have to admit seldom praying for government leaders regarding marijuana laws and policy.

CHRISTIAN PHYSICIANS SHOULD OPERATE AT A HIGHER STANDARD

According to James 3, leaders and teachers will give an account and be judged more strictly concerning their words and deeds. Since physicians are leaders and teachers de facto, they must be careful never to abuse or neglect that authority. They should consider taking a public stand against medical marijuana by educating and informing those in their churches and communities.

Finally, Christian physicians should patiently and compassionately listen to the sufferings that are driving patients to ask them for marijuana, as they are hurting in some fashion. After listening carefully, physicians need to be courageous and go against public opinion by steering patients away from medical marijuana and toward truthful and honest research.

KEY POINTS

Never before has a substance been legalized as "medicine" by popular vote.

Medicines are tested for safety, side effects and potential interactions with other drugs before they are given to the general public. Medicines are tested at various doses for specific ailments before physicians recommend them to patients. Precisely regulated production and distribution channels are established before medicines are made available to pharmacists. Physicians are educated before they prescribe.

Medical marijuana has not passed any of these tests. Instead, these laws subject millions to fraudulent health claims and potentially dangerous self-treatment.

Healthcare professionals and patients should be discouraging the approval and use of marijuana for medical purposes while, at the same time, advocating for additional research into the potential health benefits of substances in the plant. Medical illnesses are best treated with FDA-approved pharmaceutical-grade medications.

CITATIONS

1   Compassionate Certification Centers. List of Qualifying Health Conditions for Medical Marijuana in Each State. October 26, 2017. *https://www.compassionatecertification-centers.com/list-of-qualifying-health-conditions-for-medical-marijuana-in-each-state/*
2   National Academies of Sciences Engineering and Medicine. The Health Effects of Cannabis and Cannabinoids: The Current State of Evidence and Recommendations for Research. Washington, DC: The National Academies Press; 2017.

3   *https://www.ajc.com/news/national/such-thing-medical-marijuana-health-secretary-says/eZkOYR0zXTghh1seUvQPAI/*

4   *https://m.youtube.com/watch?v=YeVs7aTh9vw*

5   *https://www.drugabuse.gov/publications/drugfacts/marijuana-medicine*

6   *https://newsroom.clevelandclinic.org/2019/01/10/why-cleveland-clinic-wont-recommend-medical-marijuana-for-patients/*

7   *https://www.hhs.gov/surgeongeneral/reports-and-publications/addiction-and-substance-misuse/advisory-on-marijuana-use-and-developing-brain/index.html*

8   Ebbert J et al., "Medical Cannabis," *Mayo Clinic Proceedings* 2018; 93(12):1842-1847.

9   Cort B, *Weed Inc: The truth about the THC, the pot lobby, and the commercial marijuana industry.* Deerfield Beach, Florida: Health Communications; 2017.

10 Braun IM, Wright A, Peteet J, et al., "Medical Oncologists' Beliefs, Practices, and Knowledge Regarding Marijuana Used Therapeutically: A Nationally Representative Survey Study," *J Clin Oncol* 2018; 36(19): 1957-62.

11 Kleber HD, Dupont, RL, "Physicians and Medical Marijuana," *American Journal of Psychiatry* 2012;169(6).

12 Hill K, *Marijuana: The Unbiased Truth About the World's Most Popular Weed.* Center City, Minnesota: Hazelden Publishing; 2015.

13 *https://www.washingtonpost.com/local/md-politics/amid-talk-of-legalization-marylands-medical-cannabis-industry-expands/2019/09/08/a33a1afe-cfee-11e9-8c1c-7c8ee785b855_story.html*

14 *https://www.wsj.com/articles/if-weed-is-medicine-so-is-budweiser-11547770981*

15 *https://www.npr.org/templates/story/story.php?storyId=123570215*

16 Paschall MJ, Grube JW, Biglan A, "Medical marijuana legalization and marijuana use among youth in Oregon," *The Journal of Primary Prevention* 2017; 38(3): 329-41.

17 Hasin DS, Sarvet AL, Cerda M, et al., "US Adult Illicit Cannabis Use, Cannabis Use Disorder, and Medical Marijuana Laws 1991-1992 to 2012-2013," *JAMA Psychiatry* 2017; 74(6): 579-88.

18 Tashkin DP, "Effects of marijuana smoking on the lung," *Ann Am Thorac Soc* 2013;10(3):239-247.

19 Owen KP, Sutter ME, Albertson TE, "Marijuana: respiratory tract effects," *Clin Rev Allergy Immunol* 2014;46(1):65-81.

20 Hancox RJ, Poulton R, Ely M, et al., "Effects of cannabis on lung function: a population-based cohort study," *Eur Respir J* 2010;35(1):42-47.

CHAPTER 10

The Legalization of Recreational Marijuana

"We should also recognize legalization for what it is: the large-scale commercialization and marketing of an addictive—and therefore highly profitable—substance…In states that have legalized, youth marijuana use now exceeds the national average, the black market continues to thrive and employers struggle with more drug-impaired workers than before pot was legalized."
—Patrick Kennedy (March 8, 2017, Washington Post)[1]

The term recreational marijuana refers to any form of marijuana used for recreational, non-medical reasons. The legalization of recreational marijuana makes purchasing marijuana for recreation—for the sole purpose of getting high—permissible and lawful. As of October 2019, a total of 11 states (and the District of Columbia) have legalized recreational marijuana despite the fact that it is a Schedule I (illegal) drug by federal standards.

FEDERAL VS. STATE

Like Greek dramas of old, the federal government's *agon* with the states seems unending, and recent administrations have done little to settle the matter. The Obama administration opted for a *laissez-faire* approach, letting states do what they want as long as they meet basic criteria like not transporting marijuana across state lines.

The Trump administration has taken a tougher and more traditional stance, allowing federal prosecutors to crack down on marijuana "excesses" even in states where it's legal by state statue. So, it's a rather confusing situation legally. Regardless, marijuana is legal and available in several states.

RECREATIONAL MARIJUANA BASICS

Legalizing recreational marijuana gives it a status similar to other legal addictive substances, such as alcohol or tobacco. In order to purchase recreational marijuana (the exact process varies by state), all a person needs to do is present a driver's license or some other government-issued identification to prove state residency and meet minimum age requirements. Some states will also process information into a computer tracking system to ensure compliance with monthly limits.

Importantly, legalization for recreational use does not mean that marijuana is treated like any other commodity, i.e., candy, soda or popcorn. If someone sells marijuana and is not a licensed vendor, he or she risks arrest. If teens bring marijuana to school, they could face sanctions. Just like public laws that restrict drinking alcohol or smoking cigarettes, the legalization of recreational marijuana comes with qualifications.

COMMERCIALIZATION GONE WILD

In states that allow recreational marijuana, the degree of commercialization has flabbergasted most experts. Market forces have increased demand, reduced prices and made marijuana available in about every form possible: brownies, gummy candies, honey, joint balms, capsules, creams, juices, sodas, coffee, beers, suppositories, concentrates, cakes, tinctures, cookies, etc. Consumer demand has led to concentrations that defy imagination. This is not the decriminalization of marijuana; instead, it is the legalization of the marketing, commercialization and capitalization of THC.[2]

INVESTMENTS SOAR

The legalization of recreational marijuana has stimulated significant capital investments in marijuana companies. Large corporations have entered the market with Big Tobacco and Big Alcohol companies leading the way. In states like California and Colorado, "mom and pop" operations are complaining they are being pushed out by these heavily capitalized formidable entities. In Canada, more than 160 of the 567 companies listed on the Canadian Security Exchange are in marijuana-related businesses.[3] (These companies are barred from the U.S. Stock Exchange because of federal laws.) *Forbes*, *Fortune* and *The Wall Street Journal* have all had cover stories on the rising amounts of capital flowing into marijuana business and stocks.[4] Now, people don't invest in a company because they like the product; instead, they invest because they want to earn a profit. When it comes to marijuana, profit requires more users and these savvy sophisticated companies will spend millions figuring out how to lure more people to marijuana. Just the idea of having powerful corporations with large advertising budgets involved in the marketing of another potentially harmful and addictive substance should worry every American.[5] Remember the Marlboro Man ads?

KID-FRIENDLY MARKETING

One of the most disturbing aspects of commercialization has been the marketing of marijuana to young people. Just like we had Joe Camel for cigarettes, we now have teen-friendly products: infused gummy bears, candies, sodas, Reefer's peanut butter cups, Santa Claus candy, Girl Scout Cooke Shatter and a cartoon character called Buddy.[6] According to a September 2019 article in the medical journal *Addictive Behaviors*, young adults aged 18 to 24 were almost twice as likely as older adults to start vaping because of the teen-friendly flavors. In an American Heart Association news release, the lead author said, "These findings are especially disturbing when you consider the many kid-friendly flavor options that entice younger users to first try e-cigarettes…that now fuel addiction to these products."[7]

SUPER SIZE ME

Packaging, labeling issues and serving sizes are an issue. The legal limit per serving in Colorado is supposed to be 10 milligrams of THC, which is an amount unlikely to lead to an overdose. So, a logical person might assume one Cheeba Chew contains 10 mg of THC. (Cheeba Chews are taffy Jolly-Rancher-sized THC-infused candies). One Cheeba Chew, to the praise of *High Times* magazine, actually contains 100 milligrams of THC or 10 servings per piece.[8] Is anyone really going to cut the candy into 10 pieces? Of course not.

Manufacturers make things like this because purposely written ambiguous laws allow them, and they get headlines in magazines and on the internet as they push the limits. But they argue absurdly that the buyer is fully informed and adequately warned because each package says, "Caution: Extremely Potent." Even the run-of-the-mill THC gummy bear contains 40 mg of THC with instructions stating "four servings per bear."[9] Has anyone ever eaten one-fourth of a gummy bear?

A WELL-INFORMED CONSUMER?

Five out of six tobacco smokers will <u>not</u> die of lung cancer. But, as a society, cigarette use plummeted among teens and young people when we told the truth and made it widely known that cigarettes can cause cancer and illness. Not everyone who drives drunk kills someone. But Mothers Against Drunk Driving (MADD) and other organizations have gotten the message out and drunk driving has been reduced. Unfortunately, we have not been honest with our children, our young people and ourselves about marijuana.

According to the *American Academy of Child and Adolescent Psychiatry*, the legalization of marijuana "may be associated with (a) decrease in adolescent perception of marijuana's harmful effects, (b) increased marijuana use among parents and caretakers, and (c) increased adolescent access to marijuana, all of which reliably predict increased rates of adolescent marijuana use and associated problems…Furthermore, marijuana's deleterious effects on adolescent cognition, behavior, and brain development may have immediate and long-term implications including increased risk of motor vehicle accidents, sexual victimization, academic failure, lasting decline in intelligence measures, psychological and occupational impairment."[10]

WHAT HAPPENS TO THE BLACK MARKET WHEN RECREATIONAL MARIJUANA IS LEGALIZED?

Interestingly, many people speculated the black market would disappear once recreational marijuana was legalized. *Au contraire*, there is evidence it has increased as consumers, looking for better prices, flocked to the no-tax, less-expensive marijuana products available outside the dispensaries. In a *Denver Post* opinion piece on September 28, 2018, Attorney General for Colorado Bob Troyer wrote, "…Colorado's black market has actually exploded after commercialization: we have become a source-state, a theater of operation for sophisticated international drug trafficking and money laundering operations from Cuba, China, Mexico, and elsewhere."[11]

The same story is true in California. A September 2019 analysis by the United Cannabis Business Association found that illegal sellers outnumber legal and regulated businesses almost 3-to-1. And that's two years *after* recreational marijuana became legal in California.[12]

An increase in the black market means millions and millions of dollars flow into the hands of organized crime, and this has offshoots into other criminal activities. Finally, the average black marketer sells an array of drugs, and a customer buying marijuana will inevitably be offered more dangerous drugs like heroin, ecstasy or meth.

ARGUMENTS FOR AND AGAINST RECREATIONAL MARIJUANA

There are legitimate arguments for and against recreational marijuana, and the thoughtful citizen should consider these carefully. I tried to list most of these in tables 1 and 2. I am not going to discuss them here in detail as they are specifically addressed in other chapters. The American Medical Association, the American Psychiatric Association, the American Academy of Child and Adolescent Psychiatry, the American Academy of Pediatrics, the American Academy of Addiction Psychiatry, the American Society of Addiction Medicine have all published position papers outlining why they oppose legalizing marijuana. You can access their rationale online.

Table 1
Arguments in Favor of Legalizing Recreational Marijuana

- Increases personal liberties
- Increases tax revenues
- Reduces law enforcement costs and time
- Reduces incarceration rates
- Reduces racial disparities in marijuana
- arrests/convictions
- Honors the will of the people
- Allows for state control and regulation
- Increases the safety of the marijuana being sold

Table 2
Arguments Against Legalizing Recreational Marijuana

- Increases the number of users
- Increases the number of first-time and teen users
- Increases the number of addictions
- Increases the marketing and commercialization of marijuana
- Increases medical costs
- Leads to social disruption of families and communities
- Increases car accidents
- Increases the use of harder and more dangerous drugs
- Increases the black market as marijuana consumers avoid taxes
- Results in premature deaths and illnesses
- Testing technology is not available to determine impaired driving

DIFFERENCES BETWEEN RECREATIONAL MARIJUANA AND RECREATIONAL ALCOHOL

Many of the arguments for and against marijuana seem to find their basis in alcohol comparisons with some saying, "it is safer" and others saying, "it is more dangerous." It's like comparing apples with oranges in some sense, as alcohol and marijuana are consumed differently, metabolized differently and have different short-term and long-term effects. But I do think a head-to-head juxtaposition can be enlightening.

1.   **The moderate use of marijuana is uncommon when compared with alcohol.**

The number of Americans who use cannabis *heavily* is soaring. In 2006, about three million Americans reported using cannabis at least 300 times a year. By 2017, that number had nearly tripled to eight million.[13]

Dr. Kevin Hill, an assistant professor of psychiatry at Harvard's McLean Hospital, explains in his 2015 book that alcohol use is spread out fairly even in the population—resembling a nice bell curve distribution—from teetotalers to problem drinkers with lots of people in the middle.[5] Most people who use marijuana, on the other hand, use it rarely (socially) or frequently; as a result, it's a biphasic distribution pattern with only a few people in the middle. Only one in 15 drinkers consumes alcohol daily, but one in five marijuana users takes cannabis daily.[5,13]

When interviewed, people who have tried marijuana will generally tell you they either liked the way it made them feel, or they didn't. In other words, the moderate use of marijuana is less common than with alcohol. Therefore, it is dangerous and naive for people to assume they can limit their usage like so many people limit their daily use of alcohol.

2.   **Daily use of marijuana is considered heavy use.**

Using marijuana daily or nearly daily (more than 300 times a year) is the level at which it typically starts affecting work and school performance, relationships and personality.[9] That is not the situation for a daily glass of wine.

3.   **It's more difficult to control the dose of marijuana or degree of impairment.**

The strengths of various alcohol preparations are well-established and standardized. With alcohol, it takes at least two drinks in order to feel the effects, and hardly anyone will feel impaired after one drink. That is not the case for marijuana. One or two "hits" from a joint or bong or blunt (see glossary) will usually cause some impairment. In fact, a typical smoking session might only be two hits of marijuana at a time. Given the variations in marijuana strains and potency, the degree of impairment is hard to control, especially for less experienced users.

4.   **Addiction rates are lower for marijuana.**

One in 11 adults (9%) who use marijuana will develop a substance use disorder, while it's one in seven (15%) for alcohol. One in six (17%) teens who use marijuana will develop a substance use disorder. However, teen marijuana users progress to more addictive and harder drugs more frequently than teens who consume alcohol.

5. **The only goal of marijuana is to get high.**

    As one of my friends likes to say, "You don't pair marijuana with chicken." In other words, the sole purpose of marijuana is to get high. That is not true of a glass of wine with dinner. It is unlikely for a person to smoke marijuana without getting high, unless they are trying to be "social" and are intentionally not inhaling.

6. **Smoking marijuana is bad for the lungs, and alcohol is bad for the liver.**

    Both have negative impacts on physical health. Excessive alcohol is bad for the liver, but any smoking is bad for your lungs as smoking is a harmful and dangerous way to consume any substance.[14,15,16]

7. **Recreational marijuana is illegal in the vast majority of states.**

    Alcohol is legal in all 50 states, while recreational marijuana is not. For those who consider obeying the law to be a societal good and the basic responsibility of a good citizen, legality should make a difference.

MY POSITION ON THE LEGALIZATION OF RECREATIONAL MARIJUANA

I oppose the legalization of recreational marijuana for the following reasons:

1. It commercializes marijuana, which means there will be more businesses strategizing ways to increase the number of users (see chapters 3 and 4).
2. It capitalizes and monetizes marijuana, prompting large companies to move into the space creating powerful and influential promoters.
3. It creates perverse incentives whereby states have a vested interest in heightened sales to grow tax revenues, which is similar to their advertising of lottery tickets (see chapter 4).
4. It boosts the number of first-time users, teen users and use by young people.
5. It significantly increases the amount of marijuana consumed by existing users (i.e., heavy users).
6. It hurts the poor and disadvantaged disproportionately (see chapter 17).
7. It makes our roads less safe (increase in fatal car accidents, 70% of users admitting to driving when high, see chapter 15).
8. It endangers the mental and physical health of more users (see chapters 7 and 15).
9. It harms the unborn and breast-fed infants (see chapter 23).

10. It bumps up the number of emergency room visits and medical costs (see chapters 15, 19 and 20).
11. It hurts the environment (see chapter 22).
12. It increases accidental ingestions by infants and children (see chapter 24).
13. It exacerbates the number of people addicted to marijuana (see chapters 12 and 16).

In other words, the legalization of recreational marijuana has proven to be more harmful than good. In many ways, we are simply repeating the negative aspects of our history with nicotine and alcohol—addictions, premature deaths, social disruption, driving under the influence, etc. I believe the adverse consequences of these imprudent and temerarious laws will be suffered for generations.

MY RECOMMENDATIONS

1. Vote "No" on all recreational marijuana referendums.
2. If you live in a state where recreational marijuana has been legalized, encourage lawmakers to apply the lessons learned from alcohol and nicotine and rewrite recreational marijuana laws.
   a. Limit THC to under 15%.
   b. Institute a massive public campaign to educate the public about the risks of marijuana to teens, pregnant woman, young people, driving, etc.
   c. Develop programs to prevent driving while intoxicated.
   d. Restrict advertising (as with tobacco and alcohol), including advertising on the internet.
   e. Protect consumers from false marketing and disinformation campaigns.
   f. Outlaw teen-directed products.
   g. Regulate marijuana dispensaries.
   h. Develop robust strategies to prevent access and availability to vulnerable populations.
   i. Increase punishment for those selling cannabis to teens and young adults.
   j. Mandate proper labeling.
   k. Promote laws and enforcement to keep marijuana smoking out of the public space.
3. If you live in a state where recreational marijuana has been legalized, put pressure on lawmakers to reverse course on recreational marijuana.
4. Refrain from using recreational marijuana yourself, even if legalized, and take a vocal position against the legalization of recreational marijuana.

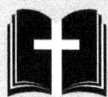

THE CHRISTIAN PERSPECTIVE
CHRISTIAN LIBERTY: WISE, GOOD, FAITHFUL AND RIGHTEOUS

I believe one of the most important things we can do as mature Christians is fully embrace the concept of Christian liberty. Instead of asking if something is right or wrong, we should be asking ourselves three questions:

1. Is _____ "wise" or "unwise" based on biblical principles?

2. Is _____ being a "faithful servant" or an "unfaithful servant?"

3. Is _____ befitting a person who is an adopted child of God?

These three questions are important when we think about topics such as marijuana, because no explicit biblical texts mention cannabis. Similarly, the Bible never says pornography is wrong, but that inference is consistent with Jesus' assertion that "...everyone who looks at a woman with lustful intent has already committed adultery with her in his heart" (Matthew 5:28, ESV).

In short, the Bible gives us a system of values and principles to help us know and make God-pleasing choices. We can also think of "God-pleasing choices" as "good choices," "wise choices," "faithful choices" and "righteous choices." In his classic book *On Friendship*, the great Roman philosopher Cicero says wisdom and goodness are one.

WHAT DOES THE BIBLE SAY ABOUT ALCOHOL?

In the ancient world, wine was the most common alcoholic drink—the prevailing recreational substance likely to cause intoxication and addiction. While alcohol and marijuana have some clear-cut differences, as we discussed above, contrasting them can be helpful as we consider biblical values and principles.

The Bible lists wine as a gift from God in Psalm 104:14-15 and other verses: "You cause the grass to grow for the livestock and plants for man to cultivate, that he may bring forth food from the earth and wine to gladden the heart of man, oil to make his face shine and bread to strengthen man's heart" (ESV).

Yet, numerous Bible verses label drunkenness as a sin and an undesirable behavior:

- "Be not among drunkards or among gluttonous eaters of meat, for the drunkard and the glutton will come to poverty..." (Proverbs 23:20-21, ESV).

- "The acts of the sinful nature are obvious: sexual immorality, impurity and debauchery; idolatry and witchcraft; hatred, discord, jealousy, fits of rage, selfish ambition, dissensions, factions and envy; drunkenness, orgies, and the like. I warn you, as I did before, that those who live like this will not inherit the kingdom of God" (Galatians 5:19-21, NIV 1984).

- Instructions to church leaders: "Do not get drunk on wine, which leads to debauchery. Instead, be filled with the Spirit" (Ephesians 5:18, NIV 1984). (1 Timothy 3:2-3 and Titus 1:7 are similar.)

The Bible is an interconnected whole, so we cannot take one or two verses and claim it is a biblical principle. I think even the most casual reader of the above snippets will conclude that the Bible's view on alcohol is nuanced. Alcohol is a categorical good but prone to misuse and abuse.

Virtually everyone has a family member or friend whose life was ruined by alcohol. The misuse and abuse of alcohol has led to much human suffering: joblessness, crime, fatal auto accidents, liver disease, physical violence, domestic abuse, sexual violence, financial difficulties, family strain, premature death, divorce, etc. A list like this makes it seem reasonable for many people—including many Christians—to choose not to drink and to preach against it. Yet, given the positive verses outlined above, it seems untenable to conclude that the Bible prohibits alcohol.

When used in moderation, the Bible says wine is good in the way it cheers people, fosters relationships and enhances community events like weddings. It's even promised in heaven (Mark 14:25, Isaiah 25:6 and Luke 22:18). And since Jesus drank wine, those wearing "What Would Jesus Do" bracelets will have a hard time opposing all alcohol.

The Bible is also clear that drinking to excess fails our test of wise, faithful and righteous conduct. The Bible views drunkenness as an undesirable behavior, and it also lists many of the specific troubles and ills alcohol can bring to the individual, family and society. Finally, while we have full liberty under Christ, we are told to not be mastered by or addicted to anything and to always consider how our behavior will affect others (1 Corinthians 6:12).

THE SAME BIBLICAL VALUES AND PRINCIPLES APPLY

I believe many of these same values and principles we applied to alcohol can be applied to marijuana. We should avoid drunkenness (getting high). We should avoid behaviors that can lead to a substance use disorder. But, what about a low-level use of marijuana? Shouldn't that be ok? What's the difference between a glass of wine with dinner and a joint after work? I believe we have answered that question above, but let's overlay it onto the Christian worldview.

APPLYING THE PRINCIPLES TO MARIJUANA

1. **The moderate use of marijuana is rare.**

   It is dangerous and naive for Christians to assume they can limit their usage of marijuana in the same way many Christians limit their daily use of alcohol. We are warned to not be mastered by anything in 1 Corinthians 6:12. In addition, it is much harder with marijuana to control the degree of impairment, and the Bible cautions us about drunkenness or getting high.

2. **Daily use is considered high use.**

   Smoking a joint daily is the level at which marijuana typically starts affecting work and school performance, relationships and personality. In other words, it can hamper believers from fulfilling their God-ordained purposes at home, work and church. That is not the situation for a daily glass of wine.

3. **Recreational marijuana is illegal in the vast majority of states.**

   If it's illegal, Christians shouldn't do it unless the law violates a higher principle (Romans 13:1-7).

4. **The use of recreational marijuana may adversely affect others.**

   "Everyone should look out not only for his own interests, but also for the interests of others" (Philippians 2:4, CSB). Even if we think we are free to smoke marijuana under Christian liberty, abstaining because it might hurt another would be an example of Christian liberty beautifully serving the ends of Christian love. "For you were called to be free, brothers and sisters; only don't use this freedom as an opportunity for the flesh, but serve one another through love" (Galatians 5:13, CSB).

5.   Smoking marijuana is bad for your lungs.

As it says in 1 Corinthians 6:19-20, our bodies are the temple of God, and smoking is unhealthy.

A BOLD VISION FOR HUMAN FLOURISHING

Sometimes the prohibitions of Scripture seem harsh. Even the word "prohibition" rings abrasively. A biblical view of alcohol (our best corollary for marijuana) feels defensive and negative. But the commands of the Bible grow out of a promising and optimistic view of human flourishing—a revolutionary transforming vision of wellness and healthy relationships. It is aligning with the divine; going far beyond physical health. It is thriving socially, emotionally, intellectually and spiritually, regardless of one's circumstances. Biblical imperatives draw us to Christ with the promise of well-being and peace. "Consider how I love your precepts! Give me life according to your steadfast love" (Psalm 119:159, ESV).

RECOMMENDATIONS FOR CHRISTIANS

The Christian desiring to be wise, good, faithful and righteous should consider abstaining from recreational marijuana, even if legalized. We may also want to weigh taking positions against the legalization of recreational marijuana at the ballot box and in the public square.

KEY POINTS

The legalization of recreational marijuana makes lawful and permissible the purchase and possession of marijuana by adults. It is the commercialization, monetization and capitalization of an addictive and intoxicating substance that possesses medical and psychiatric risks. Using tactics eerily similar to Big Tobacco and Big Alcohol, the marijuana industry is repeating the negative aspects of our history with nicotine and alcohol—addictions, premature deaths, adverse health outcomes, homelessness, social disruption, financial stress, driving under the influence, etc.—all in the pursuit of profit and personal freedom.

CITATIONS

1 Kennedy P, Sabet K, "Don't Let Big Marijuana Prioritize Profits over Public Safety," *Washington Post* (March 8, 2017).

2 Cort B, *Weed Inc: The truth about the THC, the pot lobby, and the commercial marijuana industry*. Deerfield Beach, Florida: Health Communications; 2017.

3 *https://abcnews.go.com/International/californias-biggest-cannabis-companies-grow-green-canadian-stock/story?id=63529520*

4 *https://www.kitco.com/news/2018-01-05/Canada-exchange-asks-pot-firms-to-disclose-risks-on-U-S-operations.html*

5 Hill K, *Marijuana: The Unbiased Truth About the World's Most Popular Weed*. Center City, Minnesota: Hazelden Publishing; 2015.

6 Landry LL, Groom AL et al, "The role of flavors in vaping initiation and satisfaction among U.S. adults," *Addiction Behaviors* 2019;99.

7 *https://newsroom.heart.org/news/study-finds-flavors-play-a-role-in-initiation-addiction-to-e-cigarette-use?preview=9115*

8 *https://hightimes.com/business/a-look-inside-the-cheeba-chews-candy-factory/*

9 Cort B, *Weed Inc: The truth about the THC, the pot lobby, and the commercial marijuana industry*. Deerfield Beach, Florida: Health Communications; 2017.

10 *https://www.aacap.org/AACAP/Policy_Statements/2014/aacap_marijuana_legalization_policy.aspx*

11 *https://www.denverpost.com/2018/09/28/colorado-marijuana-commercialization/*

12 *https://www.latimes.com/california/story/2019-09-11/california-marijuana-black-market-dwarfs-legal-pot-industry*

13 Berenson, A; *Tell Your Children: The Truth About Marijuana, Mental Illness and Violence*. Glencoe, Illinois: Free Press; 2018.

14 Tashkin DP, "Effects of marijuana smoking on the lung," *Ann Am Thorac Soc* 2013;10(3):239-247.

15 Owen KP, Sutter ME, Albertson TE, "Marijuana: respiratory tract effects," *Clin Rev Allergy Immunol* 2014;46(1):65-81.

16 Hancox RJ, Poulton R, Ely M, et al., "Effects of cannabis on lung function: a population-based cohort study," *Eur Respir J* 2010;35(1):42-47.

CHAPTER 11

Decriminalization of Marijuana

"Communities of color have been disproportionately impacted by laws governing marijuana for far too long, and today we are ending this injustice once and for all. By providing individuals who have suffered the consequences of an unfair marijuana conviction with a path to have their records expunged and by reducing draconian penalties, we are taking a critical step forward in addressing a broken and discriminatory criminal justice process."
—Governor of New York Andrew Cuomo, commenting on the passage of the New York State decriminalization law (July 29, 2019)

More than 23 states and the District of Columbia have decriminalized marijuana. Decriminalization establishes possession of marijuana as a civil offense rather than a criminal offense. Its goal is to maintain a commensurate deterrent (a fine) for users while focusing law enforcement on growers, distributors and sellers.

Decriminalization is vastly different from legalization. When legalized, marijuana is treated like alcohol and cigarettes, which means it is subject to regulations

Decriminalization is an attempt to focus law enforcement on the producers, distributors and sellers, rather than on the users.

but completely permissible and lawful.[1] Under decriminalization, the production, transportation, growing, selling and buying remain criminal activities, but the possession of marijuana has been downgraded to a civil offense.

CIVIL VS. CRIMINAL OFFENSE

A civil offense is a violation of an administrative matter. Civil offenses range from a breach of contract to violation of a noise ordinance to an individual being charged with a traffic ticket. For example, a speeding violation is a civil offense; as a result, people receive warnings, tickets or required court appearances. As with speeding, a person caught possessing marijuana may be given a warning, required to pay a fine or required to take an educational class in drug abuse. In contrast, criminal offenses result in arrest, a jail sentence and a permanent criminal record.

In the New York State Decriminalization Law (2019), the fine is $50 for possession of less than one ounce of marijuana and $200 for amounts between one and two ounces. Possessing larger amounts of marijuana, growing, distributing, selling and buying all remain criminal offenses.[2]

DECRIMINALIZATION AS A STRATEGY, NOT A DESTINATION

In the 1990s and early 2000s, marijuana advocates considered decriminalization a strategic path to full legalization of recreational marijuana. This strategy was not overly effective because the "transition mindset" created an environment that ensured its failure as a public policy. Viewing decriminalization as a transitional phase inhibited law enforcement from finding and prosecuting growers, distributors and sellers. It created a "wild wild west" mentality from growers to sellers to users. It also ensured the transition to legalization as people logically reasoned, "We might as well get some tax revenue since people are growing, selling, buying and using it anyway." Decriminalization, as a strategy, has largely been replaced by the more successful "medical marijuana strategy."

ARGUMENTS FOR THE DECRIMINALIZATION OF MARIJUANA

Proponents say decriminalization reduces unnecessary, excessive and expensive incarcerations for possession while still maintaining some deterrence. This frees up an overcrowded court and jail system and eliminates the stigma on those who are convicted, removing a possible obstacle to employment.

Supporters of decriminalization believe a fine is a more appropriate penalty, arguing the resources, time and money spent on policing individual behavior is imprudent and poor stewardship. Misdemeanor marijuana arrests in the state of New York made up 8.5% of all the state's misdemeanor arrests in 2017, consuming valuable police and court resources.[3]

Decriminalization also avoids the commercialization, capitalization, monetization and state endorsement of marijuana. This reduces the large capital investments, advertising and marketing that drives much of the increased use associated with legalization. Finally, decriminalization, because of the fines imposed, discourages the use of marijuana in public spaces when compared with legalization.

ARGUMENTS AGAINST THE DECRIMINALIZATION OF MARIJUANA

Decriminalization will probably increase demand compared to places where marijuana is currently illegal by removing the criminal charge deterrent. People who were concerned about arrest might be less concerned about a fine. Therefore, compared to states where it is currently illegal, decriminalization will increase availability and accessibility. This leads us an inescapable conclusion: decriminalization will increase access and usage by young people and other vulnerable populations.[4]

Because of the increased demand, decriminalization will undoubtedly fuel the underground market for marijuana. This will create more expansive networks of illegal sellers and distributors, and it will increase the profits and power of illegal cartels.

Compared with legalization, there is no standardization or regulation of available products. Consumers will not have any assurance the products they buy are safe. In addition, underground sellers will often try to "upsell" customers to meth, cocaine or heroin—something that never happens in marijuana dispensaries.

Addiction psychiatrists, like Dr. Hill at Harvard's McLean Hospital, argue that most current decriminalization laws are poorly written.[4] They define a "small" amount of marijuana as one or two ounces. That's about 30 to 170 joints, which is sufficient for months of daily use. Let's be clear: anyone carrying around an ounce or two of marijuana is selling or distributing. It has a street value of $300 to $800. Our public policy definition of a "small amount" is simply not based in realistic usage amounts.

As we stated earlier, several states decriminalized marijuana with the intent of it being a stepping stone to legalization. That was clearly voiced by the Governor of New York and some New York state lawmakers.[2,5] This mindset creates an "anything goes" mentality among growers, sellers, buyers and users, thereby undermining the restraint side of decriminalization.

EXPUNGEMENT LAWS

The most agreeable part of the 2019 New York Decriminalization bill is the automatic expungement of minor (low level) marijuana-only crimes. Expungement means all records of an arrest and court proceedings are removed from the public record, and the individual may legally deny or fail to acknowledge ever having been arrested for or charged with the crime. Although controversial, as there are good arguments on both sides, I see this as a fair-minded achievement. It acknowledges and corrects unforgiving penalties and the racial disparities that resulted from harsh marijuana laws and uneven enforcement of them.

Some people feel the expungement law is not needed as prison sentences for marijuana-only violations are rare. For instance, in 2017 in the state of New York, marijuana made up 0.003% of non-youthful offender felony prison sentences (usually repeat offenders or those with large amounts in their possession), and there were no youthful offender prison sentences.[3]

MY OPINION

Decriminalization, if properly implemented, could create a tolerable balance as it maintains the illegality of marijuana by having a mild deterrence, while also preventing the commercialization, capitalization and state endorsement of marijuana. At the same time, it also reduces unnecessary arrests and incarcerations.

Decriminalization has the potential to work *only if* lawmakers, law enforcement and citizens view it as a change in enforcement strategies and not as an open door to wanton lawlessness. Decriminalization should include aggressive campaigns against growers, distributors and sellers. Given the well-documented harm to teens and young people, harsh penalties should be in place for anyone selling marijuana to minors.

However, decriminalization is worrisome because it will undoubtedly increase demand, accessibility and availability. The rising demand will increase the profits and powers of illegal drug cartels. As a physician concerned with health, it is hard for me to support any action that will increase the availability of cannabis, as it will harm the health and wellness of our citizens. Increased availability means marijuana will find its way to teens, college students and other vulnerable populations.

There are no easy or perfect political or legal solutions to the marijuana issue, but decriminalization is clearly preferable to the legalization of recreational marijuana.

MY RECOMMENDATIONS

1. Vote "No" on all referendums to decriminalize marijuana, unless they come with robust measures designed to limit accessibility, availability, production, distribution and sales. All referendums should clearly outline the need for harsh penalties for anyone selling cannabis to anyone under 21 years of age.

2. Advocate for ways to fix the racial disparities and harsh penalties that have existed in marijuana enforcement in the past and present. Expungement laws for minor marijuana-only crimes should be considered.

KEY POINTS

Decriminalization of marijuana is when possession becomes a civil rather than a criminal offense. As such, a person caught possessing marijuana may be given a warning or a fine, or they may be required to take an educational class. Decriminalization focuses law enforcement on the growers, distributors and sellers, rather than the users.

Decriminalization attempts to create a tolerable balance as it maintains the illegality of marijuana while preventing the commercialization, capitalization and state endorsement. This also reduces unnecessary, excessive and expensive arrests and incarcerations.

Decriminalization has potential ***only if*** lawmakers, law enforcement and citizens view it as a change in enforcement strategy and not as an open door to "anything goes." Successful decriminalization must include aggressive campaigns against growers, distributors and sellers. Given the well-documented harm to teens, harsh penalties should be in place for anyone selling marijuana to minors.

However, decriminalization is worrisome because experience tells us it will increase demand and availability. As a physician, it is hard to support any action that increases the availability of cannabis, as this is a detriment to public health. Increased availability means marijuana will find its way to teens, young people, college students and other vulnerable populations, which is something no reasonable person should want to encourage or facilitate.

CITATIONS

1   National Conference of State Legislatures. State Medical Marijuana Laws. 1/23/2019. *http://www.ncsl.org/research/health/state-medical-marijuana-laws.aspx* (accessed Feb. 3 2019).

2   *https://www.nysenate.gov/newsroom/press-releases/senate-decriminalizes-marijuana-use-new-york-state*

3   New York State Division of Criminal Services, 2018.

4   Hill K, *Marijuana: The Unbiased Truth About the World's Most Popular Weed*. Center City, Minnesota: Hazelden Publishing; 2015.

5   *https://www.metro.us/news/the-big-stories/new-york-state-decriminalizes-pot-stops-short-cuomos-legalization-call*

Addiction, Stigma and Beyond

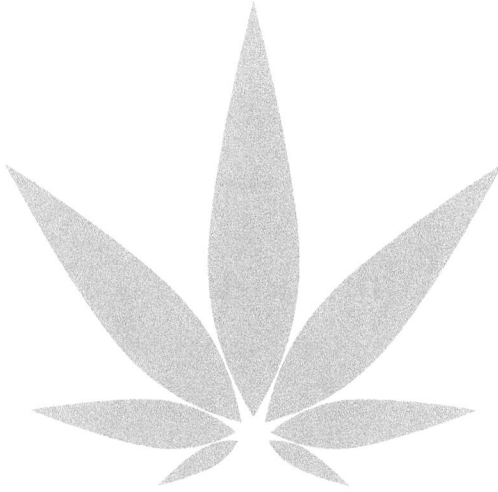

"I've had an addiction to pot from time to time. A compulsion to it. It all stems from how much pressure you're under. If you're under a lot of pressure, a joint feels so good to get off the planet that you just might decide to do it for a couple of months. I've had periods of time like that, but I don't create anymore. That's the trouble and that's what's always kept me away from going down that road too far is that I noticed I stopped painting. Figuratively, I stopped creating, and I stopped being social."

"There's this illusion out there that there's nothing addictive about it," and "the fact is anything that stimulates the pleasure center of your brain can become addictive. It doesn't have to be a scientifically addictive thing—it's a habit-forming thing."

—Jim Carrey, speaking with Howard Stern about marijuana

CHAPTER 12

Marijuana Addiction: It's a Real Thing

"He was telling me: 'Gaga you're smoking too much.'
He saved me…I'm sober now."
—Lady Gaga crediting Elton John with helping her quit marijuana[1]

In 2015, roughly four million people in the United States were found to have a marijuana use disorder. That's a number equivalent to every resident in the city of Los Angeles.[2] One in every three heavy users (daily or almost daily use for a couple of months) will, at some point, meet the DSM criteria for a substance use disorder.[3] People who begin using marijuana before the age of 18 are four to seven times more likely to develop an addiction than adults.[4]

Marijuana is not as addictive as many other substances (see Table 1) and most users will never become addicted.[5,6] But for those who do become addicted, it is a serious, solemn and trying problem.

Addiction can be defined in countless ways, but the prosaic definition known to most works well: *the repeated use of a substance despite harm or adverse effects.* Consider this oversimplified case of an emerging marijuana smoker. At first, starting to smoke marijuana is an extracurricular activity. It's something to do with friends and there is a thrill just getting some. Plus, it feels good. As the user becomes more dependent on the high, using marijuana becomes an important part of the person's life and something they look forward to. And then, it begins to slowly push out

Table 1
Addiction Rates (AR)

AR is the percentage of total users who become addicted.

Nicotine	32%
Heroin	23%
Cocaine	17%
Marijuana (teens)	17%
Alcohol	15%
Marijuana (adults)	9%

Table 2
Risk Factors for a Cannabis Use Disorder (Addiction)[3,4,5,6]

- Males
- Smokers of cigarettes (tobacco)
- Users of e-cigarettes
- Younger age of first marijuana use
- Increasing use of marijuana
- Major depressive disorder
- Younger age of first alcohol use
- Poor school performance
- Antisocial or oppositional behaviors
- History of childhood sexual abuse
- Increasing severity of post-traumatic stress disorder
- Availability and/or approval of marijuana by family and friends

other significant areas. Finally, a full-blown marijuana use disorder is present when the use of a substance becomes a priority to the detriment of other areas of life.

IT STARTS AS FUN AND ENDS UP HIJACKING THE BRAIN

Many marijuana addictions start in the teen or early adult years. Without expecting it, unwitting young people are often startled to find themselves with a problematic THC substance use disorder.

Researchers have identified several risk factors associated with the development of a cannabis use disorder (see Table 2). Personality disorders, bipolar disease, adolescent ADHD and stimulant treatment of ADHD do *not* seem to be risk factors for the progression of casual use to a cannabis use disorder.

To some degree, all addictive substances hijack the normal circuits of the brain, and THC is no exception. In a vulnerable person—either due to age (underdeveloped brain), life situations, sex, environment or other factors—THC starts to negatively affect motivation, the ability to prioritize, the capacity to function and relationships.[7,8] Because of this "hostile takeover" of brain circuitry, people with a cannabis use disorder (i.e., addiction) may do harmful things to those around them. It is important to realize that the behaviors most closely associated with addiction (and the ones that infuriate even the most compassionate) like irresponsibility, unreliability, negligence at work or school, inattention at parenting, stealing and risky behaviors are rarely indicative of a person's "true" nature. More likely than not, they are symptoms or behavioral manifestations of the disease itself. To be more specific, when a person uses marijuana daily or almost daily for more than a couple of months, it may alter the brain in ways that make THC rise in importance above other needs and desires.[7,8]

HOW TO DIAGNOSE AN ADDICTION TO MARIJUANA

Nearly all experts agree that casual marijuana users become at risk for a substance use disorder when they start using marijuana every day or nearly every day for more than a couple of months. Most people—but not everyone—will start having symptoms of a substance use disorder at this level of usage.[9] The symptoms will manifest themselves as personality changes, relationship issues or a decline in school, athletic or work performance. Unless one happens upon marijuana paraphernalia, parents, teachers, family members and spouses who are unfamiliar with the signs and symptoms of marijuana addiction will not connect the symptoms to cannabis. The crucial message is this: other life problems will often appear *before* the user and others recognize marijuana use as *the principal* problem.[9]

CANNABIS WITHDRAWAL SYNDROME: SUBTLE SYMPTOMS OFTEN GO UNRECOGNIZED

The Cannabis Withdrawal Syndrome (CWS) is a well-recognized and defined entity in medicine and in addictive psychiatry. The American Psychiatric Association lists "Cannabis Withdrawal Syndrome" in the DSM-V, which is the official list of mental disorders. The medical criteria for CWS includes both psychological and physical symptoms.[10]

The most common psychologic symptoms of CWS are irritability, insomnia, anxiety, fatigue and depression. Physical symptoms, which are less common, may include abdominal pain, nausea, sweating, fever, shakiness, chills, appetite loss and headaches. Since most users do not believe marijuana is addictive, they do not expect to experience withdrawal symptoms and, therefore, do not relate their use of marijuana to these symptoms. In fact, they often relieve the withdrawal symptoms by smoking another joint. Problem solved…apparently.

The other tricky part about a marijuana substance use disorder is the gradual and deceptive development of these symptoms. It's like the fascinating 19th century experiment of a frog in boiling water.

PETIT A PETIT, L'OISEAU FAIT SON NID

Researchers found that a frog placed in a pan of boiling water would easily and quickly jump out. But, if they put a frog in cold water and slowly heated the water up to the boiling point, the frog stayed in the water. It ended up being boiled to death. The change in temperature is so gradual that the frog does not recognize what is happening. While the results of this experiment have been questioned, the metaphor holds when one considers the gradual process of getting addicted to marijuana.

SIMPLE QUESTIONS TO ASK

One way to know if marijuana is a problem is to ask some simple questions. Do you need to smoke to make things more interesting or to motivate yourself to do mundane chores? Do you need to smoke before studying for an exam? Do you need THC in order to do the laundry? Do you need to smoke to enjoy your favorite movie? Do you need THC when attending a sporting event or visiting your favorite vacation spot? Do you need to smoke to unwind at the end of the day? Do you think about marijuana when doing other things?

DELIBERATE DECEPTION

There are other reasons why marijuana substance use disorders are not being diagnosed and treated. Let's go back to the 1950s. At that time, the Big Tobacco companies, in their pursuit of more customers and higher profits, deliberately misled the public in order to hide the truth about recreational tobacco. They intentionally concealed and distorted the addictiveness of nicotine (see Table 1) and the multiple pernicious health dangers associated with smoking cigarettes. They even released and extensively advertised a "safer" form of cigarettes—filtered cigarettes—knowing all along it was not safer. Similarly, proponents of marijuana conveniently ignore the addiction potential of marijuana and the cost of addiction to society, communities, families and individuals. Even worse, there are internet and social media sites proclaiming emphatically there is no such thing as an addiction to marijuana.

CELEBRITY CULTURE MISLEADS

Celebrities have to share part of the blame for the lack of awareness. Respected and influential celebrities, more often than not, tend to speak of marijuana in glowing or at least comical terms. Have you ever heard anyone on a late-night talk show lament that nearly 70% of marijuana smokers admit driving while high? Instead, adults on late night television are regularly reduced to giggles and gaggles at even the mention of marijuana, and a serious discussion seems impossible.

Can you think of a public personality who recently warned that one in six teenagers and one in every 11 adults will become addicted? Has any celebrity expressed concern that people with incomes under $20,000 are smoking marijuana the most?[9]

One of the few celebrities to speak out was Lady Gaga who lamented her addiction: "I've been addicted, and it's ultimately related to anxiety coping and it's a form of self-medication and I was smoking up to 15 to 20 marijuana cigarettes a day...."[11]

Meanwhile, respected medical centers like the Cleveland Clinic get little press for stating that "they will not be recommending medical marijuana for their patients" as there are better alternatives for every disease or symptom.[12] The media spotlight instead tends to shine on folks like Willie Nelson who graced the May 2019 cover of *Rolling Stone* magazine and hawked his profit-making personal brand of marijuana.

NEXT STEPS

The lack of awareness about the addictive potential of marijuana by the general public is at serious odds with medical science. The gradual and insidious development of addiction and the subtle symptoms of withdrawal all contribute to making people unlikely to diagnose their addiction. In the next two chapters, we will discuss the stigma associated with a substance use disorder and the treatment.

KEY POINTS

About one in 11 adults (9%) and one in six teens (17%) who uses marijuana will, at some point, meet the DSM criteria for a substance use disorder. Even though marijuana is not as addictive as many other substances, it is a serious, solemn and difficult problem for those who do become addicted.

The lack of awareness about the addictive potential of marijuana by the general public is at serious odds with medical science. The gradual and insidious development of addiction, the subtle symptoms of withdrawal and the addiction stigma all contribute to making people unlikely to diagnose their addiction. In addition, an intentional miscommunication campaign by cannabis proponents and social media sites further deludes an already uninformed public.

A well-funded campaign to educate the public is sorely needed.

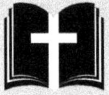

THE CHRISTIAN PERSPECTIVE
KINTSUGI

Kintsugi is the ancient Japanese art of repairing broken pottery by gluing the areas of breakage together with gold. Instead of throwing an expensive piece away, the repair highlights the brokenness and actually makes these pieces even more valuable and costly. They end up being more beautiful, but in a different way. In many ways, *kintsugi* gives us the perfect metaphor for the Christian faith regarding addiction.

Our lives are broken by human frailty (aging, diseases, anxieties), broken by personal failures (all of the times we didn't do or say the things we should have, and the times we said or did something when we shouldn't have) and broken by the suffering common to the world (floods, disasters, fires).

The golden threads of God's grace hold the broken pieces of our lives to-gether. We can be made more beautiful, by faith, because of our brokenness. Singer and songwriter Andrew Peterson captures this idea in his song "Don't You Want to Thank Someone?" when he sings: "Maybe it's a better thing, a better thing, to be more than merely innocent, but to be broken, then re-deemed by love."

George Herbert (1593-1633), who experienced deep brokenness, wrote a poem that has been cherished for hundreds of years. Simone Weil, the great French Jewish philosopher, said it was her only balm when she suffered with severe headaches and depression, and it was key to her eventual conversion to Christianity. "Love" has comforted millions because it gives hope to everyone who sees their life as a broken piece of pottery. If we are honest with ourselves, we are all insecure, unkind, ungrateful, addicted, guilty, lacking, unworthy, struggling with shame and broken.

LOVE
BY GEORGE HERBERT

> *Love bade me welcome: yet my soul drew back,*
> *Guilty of dust and sin.*
> *But quick-ey'd Love, observing me grow slack*
> *From my first entrance in,*
> *Drew nearer to me, sweetly questioning,*
> *If I lack'd anything.*

A guest, I answer'd, worthy to be here:
Love said, You shall be he.
I, the unkind, ungrateful? Ah, my dear,
I cannot look on thee.
Love took my hand, and smiling did reply,
Who made the eyes but I?

Truth Lord, but I have marr'd them:
let my shame
Go where it doth deserve.
And know you not, says Love,
who bore the blame?
My dear, then I will serve.
You must sit down, says Love,
and taste my meat:
So I did sit and eat.

CITATIONS

1   *Inquisitr.* (2014). Lady Gaga Credits Elton John With Saving Her Life When She Struggled with Addiction.

2   National Institute on Drug Abuse. Marijuana. July 2019. Accessed 9.01.19 at *https://www. drugabuse.gov/marijuana*

3   Hasin DS, Saha TD, Kerridge BT, et al., "Prevalence of Marijuana Use Disorders in the United States Between 2001-2002 and 2012-2013," *JAMA Psychiatry* 2015;72(12):1235-1242.

4   Winters KC, Lee C-YS., "Likelihood of developing an alcohol and cannabis use disorder during youth: Association with recent use and age," *Drug Alcohol Depend* 2008;92(1-3):239-247.

5   Lopez-Quintero, C, et al., "Probability and predictors of transition from first use to dependence on nicotine, alcohol, cannabis, and cocaine: results of the National Epidemiologic Survey on Alcohol and Related Conditions (NESARC)," *Drug Alcohol Depend* 2011;115(1-2):120-30.

6   Anthony JC, Warner LA, Kessler RC., "Comparative epidemiology of dependence on tobacco, alcohol, controlled substances, and inhalants: Basic findings from the National Comorbidity Survey," *Exp Clin Psychopharmacol* 1994;2(3):244-268.

7   Freeman TP, Winstock AR., "Examining the profile of high-potency cannabis and its association with severity of cannabis dependence," *Psychological Medicine* 2015; 45(15): 3181-9.

8   Avery, Jonathan D and Avery, Joseph, eds., *The Stigma of Addiction: An Essential Guide.* Switzerland: Springer; 2019.

9   Hill K, *Marijuana: The Unbiased Truth About the World's Most Popular Weed.* Center City, Minnesota: Hazelden Publishing; 2015.

10 Budney AJ, Hughes JR, "The cannabis withdrawal syndrome," *Curr Opin Psychiatry* 2006;19(3):233-238.

11 Baylis SG, "Lady Gaga Admits Having an Addiction to Marijuana," *People*, November 11, 2013.

12 *https://newsroom.clevelandclinic.org/2019/01/10/why-cleveland-clinic-wont-recommend-medi-cal-marijuana-for-patients/*

CHAPTER 13

The Stigma of Addiction

"I am me: I am not just my addiction. There is a lot of other stuff to love."
—Ryan Sachse

I remember a fellow medical intern saying (at a pub after a few beers) that he wished all the alcoholics and drug addicts in Chicago would simply die. When he saw the shocked look on our faces, he muttered, "They never get better anyways, and think how much easier night call would be."

With the insight of having many years of medicine behind me, I now see this intemperate perspective in my most gracious moments as a cry for help. He was undoubtedly manifesting the classic characteristics of what we now commonly call "physician burnout." But truth be told, my friend was also illustrating the paradigmatic signs of "addiction stigma."

The standard definition of stigma, coined by Erving Goffman, is an "attribute that is deeply discrediting" and reduces the bearer "from a whole person to a tainted discounted one."[1] In the book *The Stigma of Addiction* by Avery and Avery (2019), addiction stigma is described as having "negative attitudes toward those suffering from substance use disorders that, one, arise on account of the substance use disorder itself and, two, are likely to impact physical, psychological, social or professional well-being."[2]

Addiction stigma is a social phenomenon whereby people who use drugs are perceived as less desirable and unworthy and, therefore, can be judged and/or punished accordingly. Unfortunately, in our society, people with substance use disorders are considered fair game. That is, many people are prejudiced against people affected by substance use disorders, treat them with disdain and consider them morally flawed, weak, incompetent, dangerous and even repellent "losers" solely on the basis of their substance use disorder.

> People with substance use disorder can be infuriating. Irresponsibility, unreliability, negligence at work, inattention at parenting, stealing and manipulation are just some of the more common behaviors. But these are not the person's natural inclinations. More likely than not, they are symptoms or behavioral manifestations of the substance use disorder.

They are viewed as less pitiable, less worthy of help and more blameworthy. The blameworthiness stems from the unidimensional belief that individuals have a choice, and addiction is simply a matter of being personally irresponsible and morally weak. Yet the origin of a substance use disorder is complex and includes environmental, familial, societal, spiritual, physical and genetic factors. One glance at a person's substance use disorder diagnosis cannot possibly give anyone enough information to justify treating them in a less than whole person manner. Doing so is to be prejudiced. And if you consider that most people start smoking marijuana in their teens, is it fair to judge and punish someone for an imprudent decision that began before adulthood?

My fellow medical intern illustrated this intolerant view in his frustrating and shocking outburst. His underlying premise was people with substance use disorders have less value, are drains on society and hurt the "good" people (like medical interns), and everyone would be better off if they were dead. Let's face it, people with substance use disorders *can* be infuriating.

Irresponsibility, unreliability, negligence at work, inattention at parenting, stealing and manipulation are just some of the more common behaviors. But these are not the person's natural inclinations. More likely than not, these are symptoms or behavioral manifestations of the substance use disorder. When a person uses marijuana daily, it alters the brain in ways that make obtaining and using THC rise in importance above almost all other needs and desires. That is why work, school and relationships tend to suffer and deteriorate. But avoiding, rejecting or marginalizing people with substance use disorders will only exacerbate the disease (and the symptoms) and hurt the individual and society.[2]

And, as I have mentioned before and will repeat often in this book, one in every six teens and one in every 11 adults will, at some time in their life, meet the criteria for a substance use disorder.[3] The number of people addicted to marijuana in all likelihood surpasses the number of people suffering with lung disease, cancer or diabetes. But the numbers of those affected by addiction stigma are much larger, as it also affects family, loved ones, friends and caregivers. If we stigmatize the addicted, then we are devaluing, rejecting and excluding an incredibly large number of people.

SHAME AND SELF-STIGMA[4]

One universal emotion is common to everyone who suffers from substance use disorders: shame or "self-stigma." Spend a little time with anyone suffering with an addiction and it will become apparent fairly quickly that they experience shame almost daily. They feel shame because they are addicted, shame over past drug-related behaviors, shame over who they are and shame over what they have become. Shame and self-stigma, like a metastatic cancer, permeate their entire being, spoiling and dominating other senses of self. Identities like father, wife, son, Baptist, golfer, gay, writer, daughter, CEO, liberal, physician or Republican are drowned out by the addiction identity tsunami. In their own minds, to quote from Goffman, "they have moved from a whole person to a tainted and discounted one."[1]

Psychiatrist Curt Thompson says, "We all are born in this world looking for someone looking for us, and we remain in this mode of searching for the rest of our lives."[5] At the very least, he says, we want to walk into a room without the nagging fear and anxiety that we are not interesting, attractive, accomplished or funny enough. But a substance abuse disorder, personal shame and social stigma throw huge obstacles into these legitimate desires as they taint and distort our relationships at home, work and in the community.[5]

Sadly, they begin to take on the identity given by society, and many refer to themselves as "addicts" or "junkies." They start seeing themselves as having little value, and this has serious practical implications. Self-stigma reduces the chance they will seek help, support and effective treatment. (And please don't forget, marijuana addiction is treatable. See chapter 14.) Shame is a toxic emotion, as it drives people

> "For a long time I used to think this is a silly, straw-splitting distinction: how could you hate what a man did and not hate the man? But years later it occurred to me that there was one man to whom I had been doing this all my life—namely myself."
> —C.S. Lewis, Mere Christianity

into the shadowlands and isolated fringes, thereby increasing the risk of relapse and short-circuiting recovery. Finally, if a person allows shame to have the final say, it can drive them to end their life—even the strongest among us can fall prey to its pernicious pull.[5]

When a person with a substance use disorder starts to believe society's stereotypes and sees themselves as tarnished and no longer a whole person, recovery and healing become less likely. Instead, they hide from everyone, not the least being themselves. And what's a good way to hide from oneself? Smoke another joint, which, of course, perpetuates the very condition from which they are attempting to free themselves. It can become a vicious, downward, hopeless-looking spiral.

In "On Keeping a Notebook," Joan Didion says, "I think we are well advised to keep on nodding terms with the people we used to be."[6] She is admonishing us to be kind to our former selves and give them respect, understanding and grace. Indeed, key to the success of Alcohol Anonymous' 12-step recovery is the concept of not rejecting one's former self but drawing resources and sustenance from that person in order to live fully into the present version of one's self—a newer, wiser and more experienced self.

Here is what a college student—a daily user of marijuana—is likely to say: "It's constantly in the back of my head. I know I need to quit smoking weed. What started out as curiosity in middle school became fun in high school and is now necessary. I want to drown out the voice that constantly tells me that I am a bad person and that leads me to smoke another joint. But then the next morning I wake up feeling even worse because I did it again. I'm hopeless."

FAMILY AND FRIENDS STIGMA[7]

In addition to the person affected, family members and even friends suffer the stings of stigma. Psychologists call this "stigma by association." Family members, especially parents, are often blamed as one of the causes or even the reason the problem has persisted. Clearly, people explain, their parents must have been incompetent or negligent. Family members experience loss of respect and status. Even family members who understand they are not responsible admit feeling ashamed and embarrassed.

One of my uncles resigned as the worship leader at his church when his son was arrested for drug possession. Family members who do not share the behaviors or characteristics of their loved ones are affected by stigma and suffer its effects. Simply by association, friends also get sucked into the damaging vortex of stigma.

The most common outcome for family, loved ones and friends affected by stigma by association is isolation, a tendency to avoid talking about the person and the problem, a reluctance to seek help, increased anger and frustration with the substance user, increased personal stress and isolation, insomnia and heightened suffering. All of this, as with the person affected, results in unhelpful attitudes and builds obstacles to treatment.

And, of course, this makes the person with the substance use disorder feel even worse. They see the addiction problem as a permanent blot on the escutcheon.

WORDS MATTER[8]

Words are important. The words we use to describe our patients, even if we are only thinking those words, will affect how we feel about them and how we treat them. I don't think anyone would disagree that we all should strive to see every person with substance use disorders as a whole person who is in the throes of a terribly destructive disease and in need of help. Our language, therefore, needs to reflect that truth. Words such as "abuse," abuser" and "addict" have been demonstrated empirically to increase stigma.[8]

Researchers demonstrated this in a study when they asked clinicians to make treatment recommendations after reading a patient vignette. The clinicians were randomly assigned a description of the patient as either a "substance abuser" or a "person with a substance use disorder." Those who received the "substance abuser" vignette were more likely to recommend punitive interventions. In this book, I have consciously, purposefully and gradually been moving the reader from the word "addiction" to "substance use disorder."

All of us may want to use phrases like a "person with a substance use disorder" to convey, convince and enforce the idea that they are a whole person with a disease or disorder. We can diminish the power of shame and stigma and facilitate healing by creating a non-judgmental, non-confrontational atmosphere. Words, tone and body language are a critical skill.

CAREGIVERS AND PHYSICIANS[9]

According to Jonathan Avery, director of Addiction Psychiatry at Weil Cornell Medical Center in New York City, those in the medical community—and physicians in particular—are often thought to be immune to negative attitudes toward individuals with substance abuse disorders.[9] However, says Dr. Avery, studies have repeatedly shown this to not be the case. *E contrario*, there is evidence that as psychiatrists go through their training, their attitudes worsen. In addition, seasoned clinicians seem to have more negative attitudes than young physicians. Some experts believe these seasoned clinicians play a subconscious but large role in the development of the negative attitudes in young clinicians. This "hidden curriculum" has been offered as an explanation for the failed attempts to make fundamental changes to medical training and the persistence of addiction stigma.

And, once again, addiction stigma has practical and deleterious consequences.

Studies show that quality of care languishes as physicians view their patients with substance abuse disorders as persons of lower importance, poorly motivated and manipulative. As expected, such attitudes reduce physician empathy, engagement and personalization of care, while also leading to poorer treatment outcomes.

Numerous factors contribute to the development of negative attitudes among healthcare professionals. Most physicians do their training in large city hospitals and are only exposed to patients with severe and recalcitrant substance use disorders, so they don't get to experience those who have successfully recovered and live highly productive lives. They tend to see substance misuse as a moral failure, not a medical issue.[9] Thus, physicians, like the intern described at the beginning of this chapter, can falsely assume that individuals with substance abuse disorders rarely improve and aren't worth their time and effort.

KEY POINTS

Addiction stigma is characterized by having negative attitudes toward those suffering from substance use disorders only on account of their substance use disorder.

Considering those affected by substance use disorders as morally flawed, weak, dangerous, less worthy of help and blameworthy are common examples of stigmatization. People suffering with substance use disorders experience self-stigmatization as shame, reducing their likelihood of reaching out for help. Stigma also targets family and friends. Surprisingly, healthcare professionals are not immune to negative attitudes toward individuals with substance use disorders.

All of us need to be aware of our negative attitudes, thoughts, words and actions. We need to understand how we are subconsciously and unknowingly hampering the success of people struggling mightily with a very difficult problem.

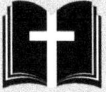

THE CHRISTIAN PERSPECTIVE
A THIRST FOR LOVE

"Homo sum humani a me nihil alienum puto."
(I am a human being, so nothing human is strange to me.)

"Then the eyes of both of them were opened, and they realized they were naked; so they sewed fig leaves together and made coverings for themselves. Then the man and his wife heard the sound of the Lord God as he was walking in the garden in the cool of the day, and they hid from the Lord God among the trees of the garden" (Genesis 3:7-8, NIV 1984).

The Christian faith is no stranger to shame and stigma, as hiding is the normal human response, especially when we experience their most toxic forms. We presume God and others will discount, devalue, reject or punish us. So, like Adam and Eve, we hide.

According to the Bible and the Christian faith, every person has a thirst for a deep connection with others, a thirst for love. But, when we fail at something, we hide and run. We run from others by acting confident, changing the narratives of our past and avoiding topics that threaten to expose our fears, anxieties and addictions. We try to hide from ourselves, perhaps by getting high, becoming a gym rat or binging on the last and greatest TV series. We all try different strategies, and some do it in more socially acceptable ways. Regardless, we all run to some degree from ourselves, from each other and from God. However, when the shame, social stigma and hiding reach noxious levels, the inevitable outcome, according to the Bible, is a psychological hell—the antipodal opposite of Eden.[5]

According to our Christian faith, the solution to this universal problem is found in doing the most threatening deed imaginable: it's called confession.[5] But we can't just confess to anybody. To use an offbeat example, it is unlikely the people who go on the "Jerry Springer Show" and confess everything under the sun benefit, thrive, feel cleansed or mature from that experience.

Confession and healing are most likely to be beneficial in the context of unconditional love—agape love. And this is something only God can offer. We get glimpses of this love from others when we receive grace instead of advice, and when we are forgiven and accepted instead of punished. Even listening in a nonjudgmental way is a shadow of God's agape love.

As we strive to embrace this divine unconditional love—proven by the cross and promised in the Bible ("If we confess our sins, he is faithful and just and will forgive us our sins and purify us from all unrighteousness" [1 John 1:9, NIV 1984].)—something miraculous occurs. The weights we carry around start to become lighter and, as Scripture promises, the truth sets us free. And then as our faith and freedom grow, they invite us and encourage us to offer the same to others so they might be more vulnerable and able to confess.

Confession is the inescapable solution because none of us can live up to our own standards. Not a single one of us can live up to the "you oughts" we self-righteously pronounce boldly and confidently to others. Most of us can keep up the charade for a while, but eventually, as we saw in the third chapter of Genesis, all hell breaks loose.[5]

Thankfully, the story doesn't end there. God seeks us out just as He sought out Adam and Eve in the garden. Adam and Eve were hiding, afraid and terrified of being known. In 1 Corinthians, Paul says, "…the man who loves God is known by God" (NIV 1984). What we seek is to be fully loved, but there is a prerequisite: we have to be fully known first. Elvis was loved by millions, but it didn't affect him deeply because he knew his fans really didn't *know* him. But to be known from the top of your head to the bottom of your feet and *still* be loved—that's life changing.

Leslie Jamison, the author of *The Empathy Exams*, sported a large wordy tattoo that said, "I am human; nothing is alien to me," when she was interviewed in the *Paris Review*. The Christian faith and the Bible claim unequivocally that shame, stigma and the desire to be loved are basic—not alien—to the human condition.

Our Christian faith tells us that all of us have a substance use disorder. All of us have failed, we are all broken and we are all full of shame. Every Christian knows we are addicted to pride, envy, greed and anger, and we need forgiveness—forgiveness from God and then we need to forgive ourselves and others.

I have been in many church settings where a person revealed a broken and especially shameful part of his or her story. I have never witnessed this type of vulnerability in any other group setting except ones specifically and artificially designed for such purposes. Of course, this takes great courage, but it also requires a safe place, a place of faith, hope and agape love. And interestingly, when shame and stigma are exposed and confessed, they begin a mysterious and powerful positive movement in those who are listening as they inevitably reflect on their own shame, failings and need for confession.

Theoretically, the church of Christ would be the place where people with substance use disorders are most welcomed, most encouraged and most comfortable. So, if Christ—through His death, resurrection and forgiveness—is the answer to disarming shame and stigma, why is addiction stigma still present in Christians and the church?

Churches do not exist in a vacuum, and Christians bring preexisting attitudes, opinions and assumptions with them to church. Inevitably, family, personal and societal beliefs influence how church members perceive and treat those with substance use disorders. These beliefs are the product of lifelong experiences.

The stated goal of Christianity is to one day see ourselves, others and our world through the Father's perfect eyes. It is a lifelong journey and process. When we see people in the light of truth, we see everyone as being one of God's children and we love them as we want to be loved. Fully. Unconditionally.

So, if that is our goal, we must start today disciplining the words we speak and, more fundamentally, the thoughts we think. Let's ask ourselves this question: are our words and thoughts reflecting what we know to be true, that God made each and every person in His image?

FOR CHRISTIAN HEALTHCARE WORKERS

You are on the front lines of care. The challenges associated with substance use disorders can bring a new openness to spiritual growth. Most of us, at some time in our lives, have pleaded, "Oh, God, help me. Show me how to live!" I believe every person suffering with substance use disorders has prayed that prayer at night when no one is around.

When a compassionate Christian healthcare worker comes alongside a person suffering with an addiction, they resist the pervasive cultural lie that this person, created in the image of God and suffering with a substance use disorder, is not worthy of care and love. They are resisting the lie that they have somehow forfeited their dignity as humans because they are weak, helpless and at the mercy of a substance. Your kindness, compassion, expert care and, yes, love underscores to those suffering with shame and self-stigma that they are not "better off dead."

A PRAYER

The following prayer was written in the 1930s by American theologian Reinhold Niebuhr (1892-1971). Commonly known today as the Serenity Prayer, it became familiar to countless Americans and was frequently prayed as people suffered through the Great Depression. The prayer was eventually adopted and popularized by Alcoholics Anonymous and other 12-step programs like Marijuana Anonymous.

God, give me grace to accept with serenity
the things that cannot be changed,
Courage to change the things
which should be changed,
and the Wisdom to distinguish
the one from the other.

Living one day at a time,
Enjoying one moment at a time,
Accepting hardship as a pathway to peace,
Taking, as Jesus did,
This sinful world as it is,
Not as I would have it,
Trusting that You will make all things right,
If I surrender to Your will,
So that I may be reasonably happy in this life,
And supremely happy with You forever in the next.
Amen.

CITATIONS

1   Goffman E, *Stigma: notes on the management of spoiled identity*. Englewood Cliffs: Prentice Hall; 1963.

2   Avery, Jonathan D and Avery, Joseph, eds., *The Stigma of Addiction: An Essential Guide*. Switzerland: Springer; 2019.

3   Lopez-Quintero C, et al., "Probability and predictors of transition from first use to dependence on nicotine, alcohol, cannabis and cocaine: Results of the National Epidemiologic Survey on Alcohol and Related Conditions," *Drug and Alcohol Dependence* 115, nos. 1-2, (May 1,2011): 120-30.

4   Matthews, S, "Self-Stigma and Addiction," *The Stigma of Addiction: An Essential Guide*. Avery, JD and Avery, J (Eds), Switzerland: Springer; 2019.

5   Thompson, Curt. *The Soul of Shame*. Downers Grove, Illinois: InterVarsity Press; 2015.

6   Joan Didion's essay "On Keeping a Notebook" can be found in her collection of essays, *Slouching Towards Bethlehem* (1968).

7   Wilkens, C, "Bad Parents, Codependents and Other Stigmatizing Myths About Substance Use Disorder in the Family." *The Stigma of Addiction: An Essential Guide*. Avery, JD and Avery, J (Eds), Switzerland: Springer; 2019.

8   Wakeman, S, "The Language of Stigma and Addiction," *The Stigma of Addiction: An Essential Guide*. Avery, JD and Avery, J (Eds), Switzerland: Springer; 2019.

9   Avery, J, "The Stigma of Addiction in the Medical Community," *The Stigma of Addiction: An Essential Guide*. Avery, JD and Avery, JJ (Eds), Switzerland: Springer; 2019.

CHAPTER 14

Treatments for a Marijuana Use Disorder

"Getting sober was one of the three pivotal events in my life, along with becoming an actor and having a child. Of the three, finding my sobriety was the hardest thing."
—Robert Downey, Jr., actor

While no FDA-approved medications are available for a marijuana use disorder, there is much we can do for the approximately four million Americans addicted to marijuana.[1] This chapter gives us an important message of hope, because unless someone personally experiences the terrible toll a substance use disorder inflicts on a person and their family, it is hard to appreciate the immensity of the struggle and magnitude of the wreckage.

THE FIRST THREE STEPS

Several levels of treatment are available for a marijuana use disorder, but the first three steps may be the hardest: (1) recognizing the problem; (2) acknowledging the problem; and (3) meeting with an addiction expert.

For most people, the best first contact after recognizing and acknowledging the problem is meeting with one's primary care physician. He or she can do a quick screening, determine if the person has a substance use disorder and then refer the person to a local professional. Referral options include substance abuse counselors, addiction social workers, addiction psychologists and addiction psychiatrists. Once a thorough evaluation is done by the expert, a course of treatment will be established.

EVERYONE IS DIFFERENT[2]

Many treatment options exist, and that's a good thing because everyone has an inimitable story. Giving people options, control and choice is important as it gets them involved and invested. Forcing people into rehab, although popular on television and in movies, might get them into rehab, but it makes success less likely. Rehab might not be the best program for them, and here's the key: it's not getting into rehab that's important, it's the mindset of the person when they leave. With the help of an expert, the goal is to try to find the best treatment plan for each individual—a person with a distinctive personality, unique needs, individual issues and singular goals. It is important to note, as well, that many (probably most) people stop abusing substances on their own without any rehab, treatment, intervention or coercion.

> "I happen to think the whole modern attitude...is entirely inhuman... Everyone would expect to have to help a man to save his life in a shipwreck; why not a man who has suffered a shipwreck of his life?"
> —G.K. Chesterton, *Fancies Versus Fads*

LEVELS OF TREATMENT[3]

Currently, there is no consensus on the best way to treat a marijuana addiction. The lowest or least intense level of treatment might be considered self-directed treatment plans. Marijuana Anonymous, which is available in most major cities, is based on the successful and proven 12-step Alcoholics Anonymous program. Most people find Marijuana Anonymous helpful as they get to talk with others who understand the reality and struggle of marijuana addiction and have experienced success. It has been my impression that people struggling with a marijuana substance use disorder feel isolated and alienated from a society where most people do not even believe a person can be addicted to cannabis. They need validation, encouragement, fellowship and hope. Marijuana Anonymous provides all of these. If a Marijuana Anonymous program is unavailable (there isn't one in my small town), Alcoholics Anonymous or Narcotics Anonymous are both good substitutes.

While Marijuana Anonymous works for some (especially during recovery), most people with a substance use disorder will need a more structured and formal approach. There are numerous outpatient treatment options ranging from group therapy to individual therapy to intensive outpatient programs. These intensive programs meet three to five times a week for three to five hours at a time. They usually combine a mix of group and individual therapy.

The most comprehensive and intensive treatment options are inpatient rehabilitation programs or residential programs. These programs can be short-term (two to four weeks) or long-term (one to three months) and are usually not geared to marijuana-only addictions. Long-term residential programs might be best when significant home, surroundings, friends or family issues could sabotage treatment.

TYPES OF TREATMENT[4]

In all of the levels listed above, trained specialists have a myriad of specific behavioral interventions at their disposal, including cognitive behavioral therapy[5,6], contingency management[7], multidimensional family therapy[5], motivational enhancement therapy[6,8] and motivational interviewing. In the excellent book *Beyond Addiction*, the authors describe a holistic family approach option, Community Reinforcement and Family Training.[2] The most important factors predicting success are individual motivation, the establishment of a trusting relationship, the intensity of the therapy and the duration of a comprehensive treatment plan.[3]

MEDICATIONS[3]

It is unreasonable and myopic to expect a medication to cure a problem as psychologically, socially, spiritually and physically complex as a marijuana use disorder. But sometimes medications are needed as *part* of a comprehensive treatment plan.

It is helpful, at times, to think of addiction as a chronic medical illness like diabetes, heart disease or high blood pressure. Addiction, although different in some ways, shares many important characteristics with these diseases. For instance, medications don't "cure" any of the diseases I mentioned; instead, they control the illness so the person can have a better quality of life. Similarly, medications won't cure an addiction to marijuana. The goal is to prescribe medications that can help a person wrestling with a marijuana use disorder to function better and have an improved quality of life while addressing the underlying issues.

As mentioned earlier, there are no FDA-approved medications for the treatment of marijuana, but this is an active area of research. In the meantime, physicians use prescription medications to help people with this disorder "off-label." In opioid and nicotine addictions, the use of agonist medications has proven to be quite effective. "Agonists" provide some effects resembling the drug of abuse but usually don't provide the same high as they are not as potent. Examples of this strategy are seen when physicians recommend the nicotine patch for people trying to quit smoking cigarettes and when addiction psychiatrists use buprenorphine to help people with opioid addictions. Similarly, an article published in late 2019 in the *Journal of the American Medical Association* suggests that cannabinoid agonist can reduce cannabis use.[8]

Because insomnia is a conspicuous and especially bothersome aspect of cannabis withdrawal, some physicians are investigating the effectiveness of sleep medications. Anti-seizure drugs, nutritional supplements, FAAH inhibitors and allosteric modulators are all being actively explored.

CO-OCCURRING DISORDERS AND MEDICATIONS

People with marijuana use disorders may have other problems such as depression, anxiety, insomnia, attention deficit disorder, obsessive compulsive disease and other mental illnesses.[9] They may also have other substance use disorders, with nicotine, alcohol and cocaine being the most common. These problems will need to be addressed—sometimes with medications—while simultaneously addressing the marijuana addiction. Once again, a combination of behavioral therapies and medications works best. This topic is addressed comprehensively in a book entitled *Co-occurring Mental Illness and Substance Use Disorders: A Guide to Diagnosis and Treatment* by Avery and Barnhill.[10]

KEY POINTS

Almost four million Americans are addicted to marijuana and efficacious treatment is available. There is hope for every single person struggling with a marijuana use disorder. Treatment plans may range from self-directed programs to long-term residential facilities and may include medications. Success seems to depend on individual motivation, the establishment of a trusting relationship, the intensity of therapy and the duration of a comprehensive treatment plan.

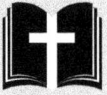

THE CHRISTIAN PERSPECTIVE
WE NEED HELP

Never one to flinch at the foibles, struggles and sins of humans, the Bible readily acknowledges drunkenness as an issue in ancient societies. It didn't look away when Noah became drunk in Genesis. More than 2,000 years later, the same problem persisted as Paul, in 1 Timothy 3:3 and Titus 1:7, was compelled to teach that leaders in the church should not be inclined to drunkenness. Paul was not arguing specifically against wine, but he was arguing against intoxication and being addicted to any intoxicant.

TRANSFORMED BY THE RENEWING OF YOUR MIND: "YOU'RE DONE WITH THAT OLD LIFE"

After acknowledging drunkenness as a real issue, the Bible recognizes the need for help at a multi-dimensional level including body, mind and spirit. In Romans 12:2, Paul talks about the need for all believers to be transformed by the renewing of their minds, seemingly anticipating our current research showing how addictive substances alter brain neural pathways.

In Colossians 3:10, Paul develops this point further by telling believers, "Put on your new nature, and be renewed as you learn to know your Creator and become like him" (NLT). *The Message* paraphrases "nature" as "life" by saying, "You're done with that old life" (Colossians 3:10, MSG). Paul was, of course, referring to the transforming new life that occurs when a person finds forgiveness from sins and discovers a new life (body, mind and spirit) in Christ.

WE NEED HELP: A LOVING FATHER WHO RUNS TO US

The parable of the prodigal son, found in Luke 15, is one of the most moving and impassioned of Jesus' parables. It is about a father who has two sons. The younger son rashly asks the father for his inheritance, takes it, leaves and then squanders the entire fortune on prostitutes and wild living. He eventually becomes destitute and is forced to return home half-starved and empty-handed. On his way back, he practices giving a speech where he intends to beg his father to accept him back as a servant. Let's pick up the story in *The Message*.

> *While (the younger son) was still a long way off, his father saw him. His heart pounding, (the Father) ran out, embraced him, and kissed him. The son started his speech: "Father, I've sinned against God. I've sinned before you; I*

don't deserve to be called your son ever again."

But the father wasn't listening. He was calling to the servants, "Quick. Bring a clean set of clothes and dress him. Put the family ring on his finger and sandals on his feet. Then get a grain-fed heifer and roast it. We're going to feast! We're going to have a wonderful time! My son is here—given up for dead and now alive! Given up for lost and now found!" And they began to have a wonderful time.

To the son's shock, his father ran to him when he spied him at a distance. He was not scorned or shunned or shamed but was welcomed back with open arms, celebration and fanfare. In this parable, Jesus is trying to show us the heart of God the Father. His boundless love transcends, overwhelms and covers our foibles, addictions and sinful behaviors. It's a story every one of us needs to hear every single day. If the God of the Universe loves us, then we can love and forgive ourselves and others.

WE NEED HELP: THE HOLY SPIRIT

In Ephesians 5:18, Paul writes, "And do not get drunk with wine, for that is debauchery, but be filled with the Spirit" (ESV). In this verse, he is invoking the power of the Holy Spirit as a helper and guide. He seems to be saying that one solution to a substance use disorder is to replace it with a focus on God and an infilling of His Spirit. This is also the teaching of Deuteronomy 6:5, "You shall love the Lord your God with all your heart and with all your soul and with all your might" (ESV). I don't think I am exaggerating Paul's point when I say he is recommending replacing a substance addiction with an addiction to God.

WE NEED HELP: A COMPASSIONATE, LOVING COMMUNITY

True to form, the Bible emphasizes the importance of a compassionate, loving and charitable community, which serves and helps each other. Galatians 6:1-2 says, "Brothers, if anyone is caught in any transgression, you who are spiritual should restore him in a spirit of gentleness. Keep watch on yourself, lest you too be tempted. Bear one another's burdens, and so fulfill the law of Christ" (ESV).

WE NEED HELP: WISE COUNSELORS AND PROFESSIONAL HELP

One of the themes of the Bible is the pervasiveness of self-deception, and our need for good friends, sagacious counselors and professional help. There are specialists who can help, and Christians should not neglect their guidance.

- "A wise man will hear and increase learning, And a man of understanding will attain wise counsel" (Proverbs 1:5, NKJV).
- "The way of a fool is right in his own eyes, But he who heeds counsel is wise" (Proverbs 12:15, NKJV).
- "Plans fail for lack of counsel, but with many advisers they succeed" (Proverbs 15:22, NIV 1984).
- "Listen to counsel and receive instruction, That you may be wise in your latter days" (Proverbs 19:20, NKJV).

GOD IS SOVEREIGN

Finally, it is always important to acknowledge and recognize that God is sovereign, and He may not take away every area of temptation or every addiction. As is well known, the apostle Paul faced an unknown thorn in the flesh, though he prayed repeatedly for God to take it away (2 Corinthians 12:1-10). As best we can tell, Paul continued to struggle with this issue his entire life. I know that sounds discouraging, and we may be tempted to give up, but we gain inspiration and an important truth when we see how God gave Paul the grace needed to deal with it on a day-to-day basis. "…'My grace is sufficient for you, for my power is made perfect in weakness'" (1 Corinthians 12:9, ESV). There is a great mystery, healing and power in this paradox.

PRAYER

The following prayer from Alcoholics Anonymous is my amalgam of the first and second-step prayers:

Heavenly Father,
I admit that I am powerless over my addiction.
I admit that my life is unmanageable when I try to control it.
Help me this day to understand
the true meaning of powerlessness.
Remove from me all denial of my addiction.
I know in my heart that only you can restore me to sanity.
I humbly ask that you remove all twisted thought and
addictive behavior from me this day.
Heal my spirit and restore in me a clear mind.
Amen

CITATIONS

1   National Institute on Drug Abuse. Marijuana. July 2019. Accessed 9.01.19 at *https://www.drugabuse.gov/marijuana*

2   Foote et al., *Beyond Addiction*. New York. Scribner; 2014.

3   Hill K, *Marijuana: The Unbiased Truth About the World's Most Popular Weed*. Center City, Minnesota: Hazelden Publishing; 2015.

4   Jafari S et al., "Diagnosis and treatment of marijuana dependence," *BCMJ* 2016;58(6):315-317.

5   Liddle, HA et al., "Treating adolescent drug abuse: randomized clinical trial comparing multidimensional family therapy and cognitive behavior therapy," *Addiction* 2008; 103(10):1660-70.

6   Stephens RS et al., "Cognitive-behavioral and motivational enhancement treatments for cannabis dependence. In: Cannabis dependence: Its nature, consequences and treatment." Roffman RA, Stephens RS, Marlatt GA, (eds.) Cambridge, UK: Cambridge University Press, 2006.

7   Caroll KM et al., "The Use of Contingency Management and Motivational/Skills-Building Therapy to Treat Young Adults with Marijuana Dependence," *Journal of Consulting and Clinical Psychology* 2006;74(5):955-66.

8   Slomski A., "Cannabinoid Agonist Reduces Cannabis Use," *JAMA* 2019; 322(12):1134. doi: 10.1001/jama.2019.14755.

9   PMID: 31550029 [PubMed - in process] National Institute on Alcohol Abuse and Alcoholism. Motivational enhancement therapy: A clinical research guide for therapists treating individuals with alcohol abuse and dependence. *http://pubs.niaaa.nih.gov/publications/ProjectMatch/match02.pdf.*

10 Avery J and Barnhill (Eds), *Co-occurring Mental Illness and Substance Use Disorders: A Guide to Diagnosis and Treatment*. Arlington, Virginia: APA Publishing; 2018.

10 Marijuana Myths, Legends and Folklores

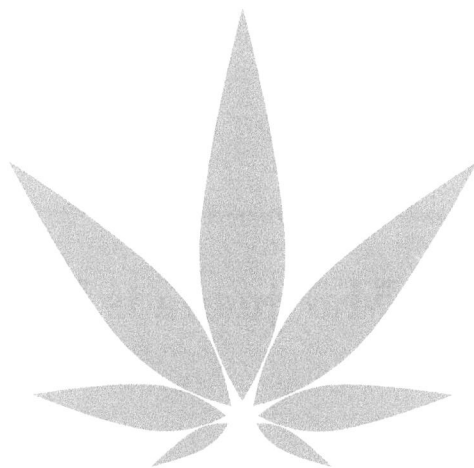

Now that we have discussed public opinion, history, botany, chemistry and biology, as well as thoroughly digested the most current medical research, let's look at the various myths and legends that have sprung up regarding marijuana. Although there is a logical order to the next 10 chapters, the myths do not depend on one another and can be read in any order, so please feel free to skip around. In order to introduce each myth properly and make it freestanding and complete, some material from the previous chapters, by necessity, is repeated.

King Arthur, the greatest myth of all time, has nothing over marijuana—fanciful stories, miraculous cures and heroes abound in marijuana circles—and many people, sadly and tragically, view them as axiomatic truths. In the next 10 chapters, we have two aims: first, to separate fact from fiction; and second, to present it in a way that is relatable and easy to understand.

"The Overarching Marijuana Myth" can be stated in four sentences: *Marijuana is natural and green and, therefore, safe, non-addicting and healthy. No one has ever suffered an overdose or died. Marijuana can make a person more creative, mellow and pleasantly high, and it may just be the answer to the opioid crisis and the morning nausea of pregnancy. In addition, making marijuana legally available to more adults will help combat social ills, improve tax bases and reduce racial disparity.*

CHAPTER 15

Myth #1: Marijuana is Harmless

"The doctors told Regina Denney and her son, Brian, what was causing his severe vomiting and abdominal pain. Neither the teenager nor his mother believed what they said: smoking weed. Smoking marijuana, the two knew, was recommended to cancer patients to spur appetite and relieve nausea. How could it lead to Brian's condition? As the months went by and the pounds slipped off Brian's once healthy frame…Brian kept smoking…Last October, after another severe bout of vomiting, the teenager died. He was 17 years old. Five months later, as Denney pored over a coroner's report for answers, she finally accepted that marijuana played a pivotal role in her son's death. The autopsy report…attributed her son's death to dehydration due to cannabis hyperemesis syndrome."
—From *USA Today* (September 20, 2019)

"I have always loved marijuana. It has been a source of joy and comfort to me for many years. And I still think of it as a basic staple of life, along with beer and ice and grapefruits…."
—Hunter S. Thompson, journalist, novelist

In this chapter, we will discuss the myth that marijuana is a harmless and perhaps even beneficial substance. After all, according to an article in the *Annals of Internal Medicine* on July 24, 2018, approximately one in every three adults believes smoking marijuana prevents health problems. About one in 13 adults believes secondhand marijuana smoke is safe for children and during pregnancy.

Even proponents of medical marijuana laws are alarmed by statistics like these. In an August 21, 2019 *USA Today* article, President of the Association of Cannabis Specialists Dr. Jordan Tishler, who is an advocate for legalizing marijuana for medicinal purposes, said, "There's an industry out there that wants to sell a lot of marijuana-based products regardless of whether it is safe or good for anybody."

SHORT-TERM AND LONG-TERM EFFECTS

This chapter functions as a reference text. I have dutifully listed most of the short-term and long-term harmful effects of cannabis in alphabetical order. Although not nearly exhaustive, I have tried to condense and summarize most of the major medical findings into this one chapter. Because of the nature of this endeavor, some things listed here are repeated and expanded upon in other chapters.

Many of these studies and the credibility of the evidence are from the NASEM report we discussed in chapter 7 but in a lengthened and more comprehensive format.[1] In this chapter, I've included study results that have "limited evidence." It is worth reminding about the evidence criteria, so please refer back to this chart frequently when reading through the potential harmful effects of cannabis. Future research will need to confirm these studies (and especially those with only limited evidence).

Defining the Evidence Criteria

- Substantial/Strong Evidence: For this level of evidence, there must be several good quality studies with very few or no credible opposing findings.

- Moderate Evidence: For this level of evidence, there must be several good-to-fair studies with very few or no credible opposing findings.

- Limited Evidence: For this level of evidence, there must be several fair quality studies or mixed findings with most favoring the conclusion or association.

The short-term effects of marijuana are obvious: slowed reaction times, lethargy, coordination and balance problems, memory issues, distortions of time and space, confusion, paranoia and elevated heart rate. Users of marijuana can get into harmful and dangerous situations as these effects can lead to falls, car accidents, poor judgment, aspiration pneumonias, heart attacks and injuries. These short-term effects are especially hazardous for those at both ends of the age spectrum: teens and the elderly.

Even more worrisome are the long-term effects of cannabis use in teens and young people. Marijuana is especially worrisome in these age groups as it is linked to a whole range of developmental, physical, psychiatric and social problems. We will list these in detail in this chapter.

ACADEMIC PERFORMANCE – IMPAIRED

See chapter 24 for more information.

Limited evidence links cannabis use and impaired academic achievement. More worrisome, this impairment appears to persist after and despite sustained abstinence.[1]

ADDICTION (AKA CANNABIS USE DISORDER)

See chapters 7, 12, 13, 14, 16 and 18 for more information.

About one in 11 adults (9%) who uses marijuana will, at some point, meet the DSM criteria for a cannabis use disorder (addiction). The numbers are more disturbing for teens, as one in six teens (17%) will become addicted. Finally, one in every three (33%) heavy users (daily or almost daily use) meets the DSM criteria for a substance use disorder.[2,3]

There is strong evidence that being a male and smoking cigarettes are both independent risk factors for the progression of cannabis use to a cannabis use disorder (addiction).[1] Strong evidence shows that starting marijuana at an early age is a risk factor for the development of problem cannabis use.[1]

ANXIETY DISORDERS

See chapters 7, 13, 19, 20 and 21 for more information.

Some individuals will experience anxiety a couple of hours after the last joint, which is known as the cannabis anxiety rebound effect. It is more common in daily users, can be quite disabling and will often persist for days, weeks and even months after the last use. This rebound effect is part of cannabis withdrawal syndrome's constellation of symptoms.

There is limited evidence linking cannabis use, increased symptoms of anxiety and the development of an anxiety disorder.[1]

ATTENTION IMPAIRMENTS (ACUTE CANNABIS USE)

There is moderate evidence linking impairments in the cognitive domain of attention with cannabis.[1] This impairment persisted despite sustained abstinence suggesting neurotoxicity and possible permanence.[1,4]

BIPOLAR DISEASE – WORSENING OF SYMPTOMS

There is limited evidence linking cannabis use and the likelihood of developing bipolar disease (particularly among regular or daily users).[1] A large epidemiological study conducted in the U.S. demonstrated a 2.6-fold increased risk for bipolar disease, along with an increased risk for panic disorder with agoraphobia.[5]

There is moderate evidence linking regular cannabis use and increased symptoms of mania and hypomania in individuals diagnosed with bipolar disorders.[1]

CANCER – TESTICULAR

There is limited evidence linking frequent or chronic cannabis smoking and testicular cancer (non-seminoma-type testicular germ cell).[1]

CAR ACCIDENTS

See chapters 2 and 6 for more information.

There is strong evidence linking cannabis use and increased risk of motor vehicle accidents.[1] Self-reported driving under the influence of THC is associated with significantly higher odds of a motor vehicle accident.[6] Cannabis increases the risk of accidents as much as 14-fold and doubles the odds of a fatal collision.

A review of 60 studies presented in 1995 at the *International Conference on Alcohol, Drugs, and Traffic Safety* found that marijuana impairs all the cognitive abilities needed for safe driving, including tracking, motor coordination, visual function and divided attention.[7]

A June 2019 survey from AAA's *Foundation for Traffic Safety* found that nearly 15 million drivers have driven a car within an hour of using marijuana. According to the AAA report, nearly 70% of Americans believe it is unlikely people driving under the influence of marijuana will get caught.[8]

CARDIOVASCULAR SYMPTOMS: TACHYCARDIA, HYPERTENSION, PALPITATIONS

High doses or use of some high potency and/or synthetic cannabis derivatives have produced the following effects: tachycardia (racing heart rate), hypertension (high blood pressure) and palpitations.[9]

COPD (EMPHYSEMA, CHRONIC BRONCHITIS, RESPIRATORY SYMPTOMS)

There is strong evidence linking long-term marijuana smoking with respiratory symptoms (cough, sputum production and wheezing).[1,10] There is strong evidence linking long-term marijuana smoking with more frequent chronic bronchitis episodes.[1,10]

There is limited evidence linking occasional cannabis smoking and an increased risk of developing chronic obstructive pulmonary disease (COPD).[1]

Surgeon General's Report from August 2019

"Frequent marijuana use during adolescence is associated with changes in the area of the brain involved with attention, memory, decision-making and motivation. Deficits in attention and memory have been detected in teens using marijuana even after a month of abstinence. Marijuana can also impair learning in adolescents. Chronic use is linked to declines in IQ, school performance that jeopardizes professional and social achievement, and life satisfaction. Regular use of marijuana is linked to increased rates of school absence and drop-outs, as well as suicide attempts.

Marijuana use is also linked to psychotic disorders, such as schizophrenia. The risk for psychotic disorders increases with frequency. In 2017, teens 12-17 reporting frequent use of marijuana showed a 130% greater likelihood of misusing opioids. Marijuana's increasingly widespread availability in multiple and highly potent forms, coupled with a false and dangerous perception of safety among youth, merits a nationwide call to action."

DEPRESSION

See chapter 21 for additional information.

There is moderate evidence linking cannabis use with a small risk for the development of depressive disorders.[1] Studies in identical twins compared those who used marijuana and those who abstained. There was a two-fold increase in depression in the twin who used cannabis.[11]

There is moderate evidence linking cannabis use with an increased incidence of suicidal ideation and suicide attempts (with a higher incidence among heavier users).[1] There is moderate evidence linking cannabis use with an increased incidence of suicide completion (death).[1]

EDUCATIONAL OUTCOMES – IMPAIRED

There is limited evidence linking cannabis use and impaired educational outcomes.[1]

HALLUCINATIONS IN INDIVIDUALS WITH PSYCHOTIC DISORDERS

See chapter 21 for additional information.

There is limited evidence linking cannabis use with an increase in hallucinations and delusions of schizophrenia in individuals with psychotic disorders.[1]

HEART ATTACKS – TRIGGERING

There is limited evidence linking smoking cannabis with the triggering of acute myocardial infarction (heart attacks), but there is no evidence that the chronic use of cannabis increases the risk of acute myocardial infarctions.[1]

IMMUNE SYSTEM

There is limited evidence linking cannabis smoking with a decrease in the production of several inflammatory cytokines in healthy individuals.[1] (Cytokines are substances secreted by certain cells of the immune system.)

There are no studies on humans connecting marijuana with an increase in infections or having adverse effects on the immune status of individuals with HIV.[1] Research in animals suggests immune dysfunction, but clearly this issue warrants additional research.[12]

IQ SCORES IN TEENS

Marijuana also affects brain development. When people begin using marijuana as teenagers, the drug may impair thinking, memory and learning functions. A study from New Zealand conducted in part by researchers at Duke University showed that people who started smoking marijuana heavily in their teens and had an ongoing marijuana use disorder lost an average of eight IQ points between the ages of 13 and 18. The lost mental abilities didn't fully return in those who quit marijuana as adults. Those who started smoking marijuana as adults didn't show notable IQ declines.[13]

LEARNING IMPAIRMENT (ACUTE CANNABIS USE)

There is moderate evidence linking cannabis use with impairments in the cognitive domain of learning. There is limited evidence that this impairment persisted despite sustained abstinence suggesting possible neurotoxicity.[1]

LUNG DISEASES

Any type of smoke inhalation (including smoke from pollution, campfires and cigarettes) increases the risk of developing lung diseases such as asthma, chronic bronchitis, emphysema and lung cancer. The smoke from marijuana is especially problematic due to pesticides, hashish oils, flavoring chemicals, fertilizers and poor production techniques.[14]

Marijuana smokers tend to inhale more deeply and hold the smoke in their lungs longer than tobacco smokers do, thereby increasing lung exposure and potential damage. However, the exposure time and harm are mitigated as the frequent cannabis user smokes far fewer joints per day compared with the number of cigarettes a tobacco user smokes.[15]

LOW-BIRTH WEIGHT BABIES (MATERNAL CANNABIS SMOKING)

There is strong evidence linking maternal smoking of marijuana with lower birth weight babies.[1]

MENTAL ILLNESS

Some research has shown that the frequent use of high potency THC can increase the risk of acute and future problems with depression, anxiety and psychosis. "Recent studies suggest that this relationship between marijuana and mental illness may be moderated by how often marijuana is used and the potency of the substance," Alan Budney, PhD, of Dartmouth College said at the 2014 APA national meeting. "Unfortunately, much of what we know from earlier research is based on smoking marijuana with much lower doses of THC than are commonly used today."[16]

MEMORY IMPAIRMENT (ACUTE CANNABIS USE)

There is moderate evidence linking cannabis use with impairments in the cognitive domain of memory.[1] Deficits in memory have been detected in teens using marijuana even after a month of abstinence.[4]

NEWBORNS REQUIRING NEONATAL INTENSIVE CARE UNIT

See chapter 23 for additional information.

PARANOIA

High doses or use of some high potency and/or synthetic cannabis derivatives have been shown to produce distressing emotional states, such as paranoia.[15,17]

Paranoia with cannabis is probably under-reported. The sheer number of jokes about marijuana-induced paranoia and the fact that dispensaries advertise certain strains as less likely to induce paranoia suggest a significant incidence, although definitive studies have not been conducted.

PANIC ATTACKS

High doses or use of some high potency and/or synthetic cannabis derivatives have produced panic attacks.[1]

PEDIATRIC OVERDOSES

See chapter 20 and 24 for additional information.

There is moderate evidence linking cannabis use with an increased risk of overdose injuries, including respiratory distress, among pediatric populations in states where cannabis is legal.[1]

POST-TRAUMATIC STRESS DISORDER – WORSENING SYMPTOMS

There is limited evidence linking cannabis use with an increased severity of post-traumatic stress disorder (PTSD) symptoms among individuals with PTSD. There is no evidence linking cannabis with the development of PTSD.[1]

One study showed that PTSD patients who were marijuana users were more likely to make less progress in overcoming their condition and were more likely to be violent.[18]

PREGNANCY COMPLICATIONS (MATERNAL CANNABIS SMOKING)
See chapter 23 for additional information.

PROGRESSION TO OTHER ADDICTIONS
See chapter 16 and 18 for additional information.

There is moderate evidence linking cannabis use with the development of substance dependence and/or substance abuse disorder for substances, including alcohol, tobacco and other illicit drugs.[1]

A January 2018 paper in the *American Journal of Psychiatry* showed that people who used cannabis were almost three times as likely to use opiates three years later, even after adjusting for other potential risks.[19]

PSYCHOSIS
See chapter 20 and 21 for additional information.

There is strong evidence linking cannabis use with the development of schizophrenia and other psychoses (with greater risk occurring among more frequent users.)[1,20]

There is limited evidence linking cannabis use during pregnancy with a small increase in psychosis proneness during middle childhood.[21]

In states like Colorado, emergency room physicians have become experts dealing with cannabis-induced psychosis.[22] According to an opinion column in the *New York Times* on January 4, 2019, "Legalization advocates have squelched discussion of the serious mental health risks of marijuana and THC."[23]

RESPIRATORY – ACUTE RESPIRATORY DISTRESS (VAPING OR DABBING)
See the Glossary for more information about vaping and dabbing.

In the summer and fall of 2019, hundreds of cases of severe lung illnesses linked to "vaping" or "dabbing" occurred primarily among adolescents and young adults. About half of these patients required intensive care unit stays and over a dozen died. The median age for the illness was 23, but the median age of those who died was much older at 50. Nationally, nine in 10 cases required hospitalization.[24]

SCHIZOPHRENIA

There is strong evidence linking cannabis use and the development of schizophrenia and other psychoses with the highest risk occurring among more frequent users.[1,20,25]

Teenagers who smoke marijuana regularly are about three times as likely to develop schizophrenia.[26]

SELF-HARM

Mental impairment and distressing emotional states, such as paranoia, hallucinations and psychosis, have caused people to harm themselves and others.[15,17,26]

SEX – IT'S COMPLICATED

Research and anecdotal evidence show that in low doses, marijuana increases sex desire and satisfaction. Using marijuana daily or nearly daily is linked to an increased risk of erectile dysfunction, reduced fertility and reduced sexual desire. One study found that 35 percent of regular marijuana users were "functionally sterile."[27,28]

SOCIAL ANXIETY DISORDER

See chapter 21 for more information.

There is moderate evidence linking regular cannabis use with an increased incidence of social anxiety disorders.[1]

There is limited evidence linking cannabis use and impaired social functioning or engagement in developmentally appropriate social roles.[1]

STROKE

There is limited evidence linking cannabis and ischemic stroke or subarachnoid (brain) hemorrhage (bleed).[1]

SUICIDE

There is moderate evidence linking cannabis use with an increased incidence of suicidal ideation and suicide attempts with a higher incidence among heavier users.[1]

There is moderate evidence linking cannabis use and an increased incidence of suicide completion (death).[1]

The risk for suicide attempts has been shown to be elevated seven-fold in regular users[25,26] and for completed suicides as high as five-fold.[26]

UNEMPLOYMENT – INCREASED RATES

There is limited evidence of statistical association between cannabis use and increased rates of unemployment and/or low income.[1]

VIOLENCE

A 2012 paper in the *Journal of Interpersonal Violence* looked at around 9,000 adolescents and found that marijuana use was associated with a doubling of domestic violence. A 2013 paper in an Italian psychiatric journal found that cannabis use was associated with a 10-fold increase in violence. A 2017 paper in *Social Psychiatry and Psychiatry Epidemiology* examined factors that caused violence in over 6,000 British and Chinese men and found that drug use—the drug nearly always being cannabis—translated into a five-fold increase in violence.[17,18,29]

One Fundamental Question

"There is but one serious philosophical question, and that is suicide. Judging whether life is worth living amounts to answering the fundamental question of philosophy."
—Albert Camus, *The Myth of Sisyphus*

VOMITING – CANNABIS HYPEREMESIS SYNDROME

Chronic marijuana use can lead to a condition called cannabis hyperemesis syndrome, a condition characterized by persistent and severe vomiting. It is often associated with abdominal pain and seems to be temporarily relieved in some patients with showers or baths. (See the beginning of this chapter.)

KEY POINTS

Over the last 30 years, medical and scientific studies have raised numerous red flags regarding the safety of cannabis. Yet over the same period, the public has come to view it as a harmless natural substance. The short-term effects of marijuana are slowed reaction times, lethargy, coordination and balance problems, memory issues, distortions of time and space, confusion, paranoia and elevated heart rate. Users of marijuana can get into harmful and dangerous situations as these effects can lead to falls, car accidents, poor judgment, aspiration pneumonias, heart attacks and injuries. These short-term effects are especially hazardous for those at both ends of the age spectrum: teens and the elderly. Even more worrisome are the long-term effects as cannabis has been linked to a whole slew of physical, psychiatric, emotional, learning and social problems.

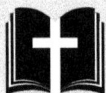

THE CHRISTIAN PERSPECTIVE
PROFOUND AND WONDERFUL MYSTERY

"Or do you not know that your body is a temple of the Holy Spirit within you, whom you have from God? You are not your own, for you were bought with a price…" (1 Corinthians 6:19-20a, ESV).

I don't think anyone can fully grasp the meaning of these verses, but the ramifications seem monumental as they encompass everything we think, say and do. This is light-years away from our common understanding of the human body as a machine, an evolved self-centered animal or a commodity. Our body is now the place where God chooses to dwell and instill His love, despite our addictions, sinfulness, lack of love, selfishness, immature faith, self-centered hopes and rebellion.

I will leave the implications of this profound and wonderful mystery up to the reader. Explore its profundities as it pertains to marijuana.

A PRAYER
Dear Father, help us to see our bodies as you do, as a holy dwelling place for your Spirit. May we use our bodies for good, to make the world a better and happier place. Grant us wisdom in our minds and strength in our limbs that we may fight the good fight, keep the faith and finish the race with enthusiasm and vigor. For your glory,
Amen

CITATIONS

1 National Academies of Science, Engineering and Medicine. The Health Effects of Cannabis and Cannabinoids: The Current State of Evidence and Recommendations for Research. Washington, DC: The National Academies Press; 2017.

2 Anthony, James C, et al., "Comparative Epidemiology of Dependence on Tobacco, Alcohol, Controlled Substances, and Inhalants: Basic Findings from the National Comorbidity Survey," *Experimental and Clinical Psychopharmacology* 2, no.3 (1994): 244-68.

3 Lopez-Quintero C, et al., "Probability and predictors of transition from first use to dependence on nicotine, alcohol, cannabis and cocaine: Results of the National Epidemiologic Survey on Alcohol and Related Conditions," *Drug and Alcohol Dependence* 115, nos. 1-2, (May 1,2011): 120-30.

4   Meruelo AD et al., "Cannabis and alcohol use, and the developing brain," *Beh Brain Res* 2017; 325:44-50.

5   Starzer MSK et al., "Rates and Predictors of Conversion to Schizophrenia or Bipolar Disease Following Substance-Induced Psychosis," *Am J Psychiatry* 2018l 175(4):343-350.

6   Rogeberg O, et al., "The Effects of cannabis intoxication on motor vehicle collision: revisited and revised," *Addiction*, 2016 111(8):1348-1359.

7   Berghaus G, Guo B. Medicines and driver fitness--findings from a meta-analysis of experimental studies as basic information to patients, physicians and experts. In: Kloeden C, McLean A, editors. Alcohol, Drugs, and Traffic Safety--T95: Proceedings of the 13th International Conference on Alcohol, Drugs and Traffics Safety; 1995; Adelaide, Australia. 1995. pp. 295–300.

8   *https://newsroom.aaa.com/tag/distracted-driving/*

9   National Institute on Drug Abuse. Marijuana. June 2018. *https://d14rmgtrwzf5a. cloudfront.net/sites/default/files/1380-marijuana.pdf.*

10   Tashkin DP., "Marijuana and Lung Disease," *CHEST* 2018; 154(3): 653-63.

11   Agarawl A, Nelson BC, et al., "Major depressive disorder, suicide thoughts and behaviours, and cannabis involvement in discordant twins: a retrospective cohort study," *The Lancet Psychiatry* 2017;S2215-0366(17)30280-8.

12   Tanasescu, R. and Constantinescu, C. S., "Cannabinoids and the immune system: an overview," *Immunobiology* 2010; 215:588– 597.

13   Meier MH, Caspi A, Ambler A, et al., "Persistent cannabis users show neuropsychological decline from childhood to midlife," *Proc Natl Acad Sci U S A.* 2012;109(40):E2657-E2664.

14   Caviedes I, Labarca G, Silva CF, Fernandez-Bussy S. Marijuana Use, Respiratory Symptoms, and Pulmonary Function. *Annals of Internal Medicine* 2019; 170(2): 142.

15   Wu, TC, et al., "Pulmonary hazards of smoking marijuana as compared with tobacco," *N Engl J Med* 1998;318 (6):347-51.

16   *https://www.apa.org/news/press/releases/2014/08/regular-marijuana*

17   Korkmaz S, Turhan L, İzci F, Sağlam S, Atmaca M., "Sociodemographic and clinical characteristics of patients with violence attempts with psychotic disorders," *European Journal of General Medicine* 2017; 14(4):94-8.

18   Douglas KS, Guy LS, Hart SD., "Psychosis as a Risk Factor for Violence to Others: A Meta-Analysis," *Psychological Bulletin*; 2009. p. 679-706.

19   Olfson M, Wall M, et al., "Cannabis Use and Risk of Prescription Opioid Use Disorder in the United States," *American Journal of Psychiatry* 2018; 175(1):47-53.

20   Arendt M, Rosenberg R, Foldager L, Perto G, Munk-Jørgensen P., "Cannabis-induced psychosis and subsequent schizophrenia-spectrum disorders: Follow-up study of 535 incident cases," *The British Journal of Psychiatry* 2005; 187(6): 510-5.

21   Fine JD, Moreau AL et al., "Association of Prenatal Cannabis Exposure with Psychosis Proneness Among Children in the Adolescent Brain Cognitive Development (ABCD) Study," J*AMA Psychiatry* 2019; 76(7):762-764.

22   *https://www.cbsnews.com/news/after-legalization-marijuana-related-er-visits-climb-at-colorado-hospital/*

23   Berenson, A. (2019, January 4). What Advocates of Legalizing Pot Don't Want You to Know. *The New York Times.* Retrieved from *https://www.nytimes.com/2019/01/04/*

opinion/marijuana-pot-health-risks-legalization.html

24   *https://www.msn.com/en-us/news/us/officials-thc-products-linked-to-vaping-related-ill-nesses/ar-AAHWN83*

25   Clarke MC, Coughlan H, et al., "The impact of adolescent cannabis use, mood disorder and lack of education on attempted suicide in young adulthood," *World Psychiatry* 2014:13(3):322-323.

26   Sums N, Horwood U, et al., "Young adult sequelae of adolescent cannabis use: an integrative analysis," *Lancet Psychiatry* 2014; 1(4):245-318.

27   Crenshaw TL and Goldberg JP. *Sexual Pharmacology*. New York: W.W. Norton & Co., 1996.

28   Gorzalka BB and Hill MN, "Cannabinoids, Reproduction, and Sexual Behavior," *Annual Review of Sex Research* 2006;17:132-161.

29   Arendt M, Munk-Jorgensen P, et al., "Mortality following treatment for cannabis use disorders: predictors and causes," *J Subst Abuse Treat* 2013; 44(4):400-406.

CHAPTER 16

Myth #2: Marijuana is Not Addictive

"Everyone is entitled to his own opinion, but not to his own facts."
—Daniel Patrick Moynihan

Steve loved playing tennis his entire life. Even after getting married and having a full-time job, he would play a couple of times a week. But when his marijuana use escalated, he reduced his tennis to once a month and, shortly thereafter, resigned from the team. In hindsight, his wife and family wish they had placed more significance in his behavior change. John would be diagnosed a year later with a marijuana use disorder in a hospital emergency room after having a serious automobile accident while high.

The huge gap between science and public opinion is most clearly seen when it comes to marijuana and addiction. Most people simply do not think marijuana is addictive despite clear scientific evidence to the contrary. As previously stated, people who begin using marijuana before the age of 18 are four to seven times more likely to develop a marijuana use disorder than adults. Plus, one in six will become addicted.[1] Among adults, one in 11 users will develop a marijuana use disorder.[2]

SEARCHING FOR TRUTH

When we search for the truth of a matter, it is best to start looking at facts, not opinions. The more facts—objective, verifiable and solid facts—the closer we get to the truth of any issue. And when we look for facts, we will inevitably seek out experts in that field. The experts in addiction medicine are addiction psychiatrists. They treat the chemical drug dependencies of patients using psychological therapies and medications. As medical doctors, addiction psychiatrists complete medical school, do an internship and residency in psychiatry, and then they complete a fellowship in addiction psychiatry. It's a long road, averaging eight to 10 years after college.

I say all that to let you know that I doubt you could find a single person in addiction psychiatry today who would say marijuana is not addictive. They see these patients every day. They hear the stories of broken relationships, wasted years, lost jobs and deep regrets—stories the public rarely hears.

Many Are Affected But Few Are Treated

In 2015, about 4.0 million people in the United States met the diagnostic criteria for a marijuana use disorder,1 but only 138,000 voluntarily sought treatment for their marijuana use.[2,3]

DIFFICULT TO DETECT AN ADDICTION

Unless a person happens to see someone using marijuana daily, finds heaps of paraphernalia or has a catastrophic event like Steve, it can be difficult to detect a marijuana addiction. While some substance use disorders are obvious, the symptoms of a marijuana use disorder are more nuanced and subtle.[4]

The telltale signs might be failing to fulfill an obligation like work or an important social event, reducing or giving up activities that were once important like favorite hobbies or church attendance, changes in personality or behavior, increased anxiety or using marijuana in dangerous or risky situations. I remember a person who worked at a healthcare facility with me—let's call her Susan. Susan was observed by a colleague to be smoking marijuana in the restroom at work. Because she was a good worker and never seemed impaired, the incident was ignored until things deteriorated, eventually resulting in the loss of her job. In hindsight, when people put important parts of their lives, such as work, at risk to use marijuana, they probably have a marijuana use disorder.

In a 2017 interview with *Vulture* magazine, Woody Harrelson talked about how he quit marijuana, "I don't have a problem at all with smoking. I think it's great…But when you're doing it all the time, it just becomes…Well, you know. I feel like it was keeping me from being emotionally available." Woody was aware enough to realize he had a problem when it was affecting his relationships.[5]

This was addressed in chapter 12, but let me repeat it again: most people who use marijuana will never develop an addiction problem. Problems tend to arise when people start using THC daily or almost every day for more than a few months. It is unlikely someone can use marijuana regularly without encountering a problem in at least one important area of life. There are exceptions to this rule, of course, but those folks are the exception.[4,6]

Some of the Signs of Potential Cannabis Addiction[1,2,3]

- Marijuana use that is daily or nearly daily
- Marijuana use that is affecting relationships, academic achievement or job performance
- Marijuana use that is affecting hobbies, personality or behavior
- Using marijuana in a dangerous or risky situation

MARIJUANA USE BY A YOUNG PERSON IS A CAUSE FOR ALARM

Let me close this chapter by emphasizing that any drug use by a young person, including marijuana, is a call for concern. The young developing brain (until the mid-20s) is especially vulnerable to addictive substances. Research at Harvard's McLean Hospital and other centers show that, among adolescents, progression from "casual cannabis use" to "regular use" to "a substance use disorder" can occur surprisingly fast.[4,6,7,8,9] And, in young people, a marijuana use disorder will advance to more dangerous drugs more frequently than in adults.[4,8,9,10]

A marijuana substance use disorder is especially problematic and worrisome in teens as it is linked to a whole range of developmental, physical, emotional and social problems. A study in 2012 of more than 1,000 people found that regular marijuana use was associated with cognitive decline, memory problems and drops in IQ scores in teens. Even more bothersome, stopping marijuana use did not fully restore functioning.[11] While this study has been challenged, other studies have documented negative school performance, risky sexual behavior, problems with memory attention and concentration, problematic social behaviors, mental health issues, increasing car accidents, depression and decision-making.[12-19]

KEY POINTS

The huge gap between science and public opinion is most clearly seen when it comes to marijuana and addiction. Most people simply do not think marijuana is addictive despite clear-cut and definitive scientific evidence.

The symptoms of a marijuana use disorder are subtle and signs will often surface in a person's life before they and others recognize that marijuana use is the primary problem. Telltale signs include failing to fulfill major obligations like work, reducing or giving up activities that were once important, changes in personality or behavior or using marijuana in risky situations.

Given the high risk of addiction, psychiatric illness and cognitive decline, any drug use by teens should be a cause for concern.

CITATIONS

1   Winters KC, Lee C-YS., "Likelihood of developing an alcohol and cannabis use disorder during youth: Association with recent use and age." *Drug Alcohol Depend* 2008;92(1-3):239-247.

2   Lopez-Quintero C, et al, "Probability and predictors of transition from first use to dependence on nicotine, alcohol, cannabis and cocaine: Results of the National Epidemiologic Survey on Alcohol and Related Conditions," *Drug and Alcohol Dependence* 115, nos. 1-2, (May 1,2011): 120-30.

3   National Institute on Drug Abuse. Marijuana. July 2019. Accessed 9.01.19 at *https://www.drugabuse.gov/marijuana*

4   Hill K, *Marijuana: The Unbiased Truth About the World's Most Popular Weed*. Center City, Minnesota: Hazelden Publishing; 2015.

5   Riesman, Abraham. "Woody Harrelson Has Quit Pot and Is Learning How to Be Quiet on Camera," *Vulture*; 2017.

6   Center for Behavioral Health Statistics and Quality (CBHSQ). Treatment Episode Data Set (TEDS): 2003-2013. National Admissions to Substance Abuse Treatment Services. Rockville, MD: Substance Abuse and Mental Health Services Administration; 2015. BHSIS Series S-75, HHS Publication No. (SMA) 15-4934.

7   Behrendt S, Beesdo-Baum K, Hofler M, et al., "The relevance of age at first alcohol and nicotine use for initiation of cannabis use and progression to cannabis use disorders," *Drug Alcohol Depend* 2012;123(1-3):48-56.

8   Chen CY, O'Brien MS, Anthony JC, "Who becomes cannabis dependent soon after onset of use? Epidemiological evidence from the United States: 2000-2001," *Drug Alcohol Depend* 2005;79(1):11-22.

9   Perkonigg A, Goodwin RD, Fiedler A, et al., "The natural course of cannabis use, abuse and dependence during the first decades of life," *Addiction* 2008;103(3):439-449; discussion 450-431.

10 Agrawal A, Neale MC, Prescott CA, Kendler KS. A twin study of early cannabis use and subsequent use and abuse/dependence of other illicit drugs. *Psychol Med*

2004;34(7):1227-1237.

11 Meier M, Caspi A, Ambler A, et al., "Persistent cannabis users show neuropsychological decline from childhood to midlife," *Proc Natl Acad Sci USA* 2012;109:E2657-64.

12 Ashbridge M, Hayden JA, Cartwright JL, "Acute cannabis consumption and motor vehicle risk: Systematic review of observational studies and meta-analysis," *BMJ* 2012;344:e536.

13 Bechtold J, Simpson T, White HR, et al., "Chronic adolescent marijuana use as a risk factor for physical and mental health problems in young adult men," *Psychol Addict Behav* 2015;29(3):552-563.

14 Bryan AD, Schmiege SJ, Magnan RE, "Marijuana use and risky sexual behavior among high-risk adolescents: Trajectories, risk factors, and event-level relationships," *Dev Psychol* 2012;48(5):1429-42.

15 Copeland J, Rooke S, Swift W, "Changes in cannabis use among young people: impact on mental health," *Curr Opin Psychiatry* 2013:26:325-329.

16 Dougherty DM, Mathias CW, Dawes MA, et al., "Impulsivity, attention, memory, and decision-making among adolescent marijuana users," *Psychopharmacology* 2013;226(2):307-319.

17 Fergusson DM, Boden JM, "Cannabis use and later life outcomes," *Addiction* 2008;103 (6): 969–976; discussion 976–8.

18 Horwood LJ, Fergusson DM, Coffey C et al., "Cannabis and depression: an integrative data analysis of four Australasian cohorts," *Drug Alcohol Depend* 2012;126:369-378.

19 McCaffrey DF, Pacula RL, et al., "Marijuana use and high school dropout: The influence of observables," *Health Econ* 2010;19(11): 1281-1299.

CHAPTER 17

Myth #3: The Legalization of Marijuana Advances Social Justice by Helping the Poor and Disadvantaged and by Reducing Racial Disparities

"Mass incapacitation of blacks instead of mass incarceration."
—National Executive Director of National African American Drug Policy
Coalition, commenting on the increased use of marijuana by African Americans
since it was legalized in some U.S. states

"We have seen the negative impact of tobacco and alcohol on our youth, families, and communities," said Will Jones, III, the African American founder of TiE DC. "Companies that produce these two legal drugs have disproportionately targeted and affected communities of color. With the costs in health care, education, accidents, lost productivity, and law enforcement as a result of substance use, Washington D.C. cannot afford a third legal drug (marijuana). Thus, we declare that 'Two is enough' and urge our fellow citizens to do the same by voting NO on (legalizing marijuana)."[12]

Despite testimonies from people like Mr. Jones, medical marijuana and recreational marijuana are now legal in our nation's capital. Certainly, marijuana businesses will create some jobs and bring in some tax revenue, but it is my opinion and the opinion of many that the poor and disadvantaged will suffer disproportionately from medical marijuana and recreational marijuana laws in both the short and long run. The few jobs these laws create are not worth the havoc they will bring on those communities, parents, families, teens and children least able to overcome the lost income, addictions, health issues and social ills. (See chapters 15, 16, 23 and 24.) The social justice argument is simply an obfuscation—a myth—so the rich can get richer on the backs of the poor. It's happened before with gambling, the lottery, alcohol and cigarettes.

THE POOR AND DISADVANTAGED ARE MORE LIKELY TO CONSUME MARIJUANA AND SUFFER THE CONSEQUENCES.

In Colorado, 20% of people with incomes under $24,000 consume marijuana products, while only 11% of those over $50,000 consume the same products.[1,2,3] For folks with less discretionary income, these purchases and addictions will exact an even greater toll on the family. Tragically, it is the children and teens of the poor who will suffer the most. It is the pregnant women in these communities, not the pregnant mom in an affluent suburb, who are most likely to consume marijuana.

THE POOR AND DISADVANTAGED ARE MORE LIKELY TO HAVE MARIJUANA DISPENSARIES IN THEIR NEIGHBORHOODS.

More marijuana dispensaries are in Denver, Colorado than liquor stores, Starbucks coffee shops or public schools, and most are located in low-income neighborhoods.[4] There is no mystery to this: people in the more affluent neighborhoods have the connections, attorneys and money to keep dispensaries from setting up in their neighborhoods. (It's the "not in my backyard" phenomena.) Poor and minority communities have fewer resources, and it is their children, families and communities that will suffer.

DISPENSARIES ARE MORE LIKELY TO BE OWNED BY THE WEALTHY.

Because marijuana is still illegal from a federal standpoint, most national banks won't finance a marijuana dispensary. In other words, someone has to put up the cash or find wealthy investors to get the business going. Marijuana dispensaries are not small businesses owned by people in the community where they are located; instead, they are owned by people of means who are unlikely to live near one of their profitable dispensaries.[5]

How Does Marijuana Affect a Person's Life?

Compared to those who don't use marijuana, people who use it frequently report the following:

- Lower life satisfaction
- Poorer mental health
- Poorer physical health
- More relationship problems

People also report less academic and career success. For example, marijuana use is linked to a higher likelihood of dropping out of school, more job absences, accidents and injuries.

Clearly, we aren't helping poor and disadvantaged communities by embracing policies that increase the use of a substance that is addictive and reduces one's quality of life.

AFTER LEGALIZATION, THERE WAS AN INCREASE IN SCHOOL SUSPENSIONS AND RACIAL DISPARITIES.

Legalizing marijuana has not reduced racial disparities for high schoolers in Colorado. Although marijuana is legal in Colorado, it is not allowed on school property. Drug-related school suspension rates (almost all for THC) have risen dramatically in Colorado high schools since legalizations. In predominantly white high schools (less than 25% minorities), there were 190 suspensions, while in schools with greater than 25% minorities, there were 801 drug-related suspensions.[5] Legalization has hurt African American and Hispanic students more than Caucasians.

AFTER LEGALIZATION, THERE WAS A DECREASE IN ARRESTS FOR ALL RACES, BUT AN INCREASE IN RACIAL DISPARITIES.

Despite nearly equal marijuana usage rates by Caucasians and African Americans, African Americans are two to four times more likely than Caucasians to be arrested for marijuana possession.[6,7,8,9]

The Million Dollar Policy Question

How do we reduce arrests and incarcerations for marijuana while supporting policies that dncrease access, availability and use?

Everyone should be concerned about the disproportionate drug-related incarceration rates for minorities. Community groups, legal experts and police forces across our country are making great strides as they reform drug policies to achieve greater racial fairness. But marijuana advocates have sharply overstated the level of marijuana-only incarcerations.[10] In the state of New York in 2017, marijuana made up 0.003% of non-youthful offender felony sentences to prison, while there were no youthful offender felony marijuana sentences for prison.[13]

Unfortunately, legalizing marijuana to reduce racial disparities in arrest rates has not reduced racial disparities. While marijuana arrests for all races dropped by nearly 95% after legalization (since the possession of marijuana was no longer a criminal offense),[11] racial disparities for marijuana arrests in the state of Washington doubled: African Americans had a marijuana arrest rate two and a half times higher than Caucasians before legalization, and it rose to five times higher.[11]

The story is similar in Colorado. Two years after Colorado legalized marijuana, the marijuana arrest rates for African Americans (348 per 100,000) was almost triple those of Caucasians (123 per 100,000).[5]

KEY POINTS

The poor and disadvantaged will suffer disproportionately from medical marijuana and recreational marijuana laws in both the short and long run. The few jobs these laws create are not worth the havoc they bring to those communities, parents, families, teens and children least able to overcome the lost income, addictions, mental illnesses, health issues and social ills.

Changes in law enforcement (and even decriminalization) are better solutions than legalization. The social justice argument is simply an obfuscation—a myth—so the rich can get richer on the backs of the poor. It's happened before with gambling, the lottery, alcohol and cigarettes.

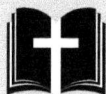

THE CHRISTIAN PERSPECTIVE
JUSTICE FOR THE POOR

When I read about powerful, influential and wealthy people promoting marijuana for profit and personal gain, Proverbs 29:7 seems prescient: "The righteous care about justice for the poor, but the wicked have no such concern" (NIV 1984). Although the sexual sins of Sodom get the most press, the Bible is clear that Sodom's most grievous action was neglecting the poor. The Bible characterizes the society as "...arrogant, overfed and unconcerned; they did not help the poor and needy" (Ezekiel 16:49, NIV 1984). Helping the poor is a Christian imperative. Paul told Timothy, "Command them to do good, to be rich in good deeds, and to be generous and willing to share. In this way they will lay up treasure for themselves as a firm foundation for the coming age, so that they may take hold of the life that is truly life" (1 Timothy 6:18-19, NIV 1984). Several verses in Proverbs make the point all too clear: "A generous man will himself be blessed, for he shares his food with the poor" (Proverbs 22:9, NIV 1984); "A faithful man will be richly blessed, but one eager to get rich will not go unpunished" (Proverbs 28:20, NIV 1984); and "He who is kind to the poor lends to the Lord, and he will reward him for what he has done" (Proverbs 19:17, NIV 1984). Christians have historically been on the front lines for civil rights, and we are and should be on the forefront of the campaign to reduce racial disparities. For millennium, it has been Christians who have helped the poor and disadvantaged have safe, wholesome and positive communities where the foundations for future success—virtues, kindness, faith, family and goodness—abound. The marijuana crisis is calling us again.

CITATIONS

1   "Marijuana Legalization in Colorado: Early Findings a Report Pursuant to Senate Bill 13-283", page 8.

2   Colorado Department of Public Safety, "Marijuana Legalization in Colorado: Early Findings" March 2016.

3   Smart Approaches to Marijuana. Lessons Learned from Marijuana Legalization, 2018. *https://learnaboutsam.org/wp-content/uploads/2018/07/SAM-Lessons-Learned-From-Marijuana-Legalization-Digital-1.pdf.*

4   Migoya D, Baca R., "Denver's pot businesses mostly in low-income, minority neighborhoods," *The Denver Post.* orig. pub. Jan. 2, 2016 updated Jan. 23, 2017.

5   Cort B, *Weed Inc: The truth about the THC, the pot lobby, and the commercial marijuana industry.* Deerfield Beach, Florida: Health Communications; 2017.

6   Alexander, M., *The New Jim Crow: Mass incarceration in the age of colorblindness*, New York: The New Press; 2010.

7   Carson, E. A. Prisoners in 2016. U.S. Department of Justice, Office of Justice Programs, Bureau of Justice Statistics; 2018. Retrieved from *www.bjs.gov*

8   Quigley, W., "Racism: The crime in criminal justice. Loyola Journal of Public Interest Law" 2012, 13, 417-426.

9   American Civil Liberties Union. (2019). Retrieved from *https://www.aclu.org/gallery/marijuana-arrests-numbers.*

10 Avery, J. "Addiction Stigma in the US Legal System." *The Stigma of Addiction: An Essential Guide.* Avery, JD and Avery, J (Eds), Switzerland: Springer; 2019.

11 Firth CL, Maher JE, et al., "Did marijuana legalization in Washington State reduce racial disparities in adult marijuana arrests?" *Substance Use & Misuse* 2019, 54(9), 1582-1587.

12 *https://poppot.org/tag/will-jones-iii/*

13 *https://ncadd-ra.org/wp-content/uploads/2018/09/Marijuana-Separating-Fact-From-Fiction-in-NYS-SAM-NY.pdf*

CHAPTER 18

Myth #4: Medical Marijuana Can Reduce Opioid Use, Opioid Overdoses and Opioid Deaths

"The claim that enacting medical cannabis laws will reduce opioid overdose deaths should be met with skepticism."
—Shover at al, *Proceedings of the National Academy of Science* 2019; 116(26): 12624-12626.

Much excitement has been generated about using marijuana to help get people off opioids. This could save lives by reducing opioid overdoses and deaths. Most of the excitement started in 2014, when a study of death certificate data by Bachhuber et al. from 1999 to 2010 seemed to suggest that states, which had passed medical marijuana laws, had fewer opioid deaths than states that did not allow medical marijuana.[1] Regardless of your view on cannabis, converting a person from opioids to marijuana must be deemed a positive because cannabis is less addictive and not as deadly.

Cannabis promoters, advocates and lobbyists touted this study loudly and repeatedly to help win passage of medical marijuana in other states. Unfortunately, they ignored the clear admonitions from the researchers to exercise caution because this finding did not prove causation. In other words, the findings did not prove that it was the passing of the medical marijuana laws that resulted in fewer opioid deaths. It could have been a host of other factors, such as changes in prescribing guidelines, physician education, the availability of naloxone, etc.

At that time, numerous addiction psychiatrists were skeptical of this study based on experience and on the fact that the United States, a country awash with cannabis, has one of the worst problems with opioids.

MARIJUANA USE BOOSTS THE RISK FOR USING AND ABUSING OPIOIDS

Skepticism seemed justified when an article in the January 2018 of the *American Journal of Psychiatry* showed that people who used cannabis were about three times more likely to use opiates three years later, even after adjusting for other potential risks.[2]

A large study was undertaken to see if cannabis could be substituted for opioids in patients with chronic pain. Published in *Lancet Public Health* in 2018, researchers Campbell and colleagues found that adding cannabis did not reduce opioid frequency or dosing.[3] Opioid use stayed the same despite the addition of marijuana. Later that same year, a study of more than 50,000 people by Caputi and colleagues (published in the *Journal of Addiction Medicine*) found that medical marijuana users were more likely to use and misuse prescription opioids.[4]

And in February 2019, a viewpoint article in the *Journal of the American Medical Association* stated, "To date, no prospective evidence, either from clinical or observational studies, has demonstrated any benefit of treating patients who have opioid addiction with cannabis." In fact, they claim the evidence suggests that "substituting cannabis for opioid addiction treatments is potentially harmful."[5]

THE LEGALIZATION OF MEDICAL MARIJUANA LED TO AN INCREASE IN FATAL OPIOID OVERDOSES

In June 2019, researchers at Stanford University found that when they extended Bachuber's study (mentioned in the first paragraph of this chapter) an additional seven years, states that had legalized medical marijuana actually had a 23 percent *increase* in fatal opioid overdoses.[6] In this study, they followed Bachuber's methods but extended the analysis through 2017. (The original study only went through 2010.) Not only did the conclusions from Bachuber's study not hold, but the association between medical marijuana laws and opioid overdose mortality shockingly reversed direction from 21% to +23%. *Namely, states that legalized medical marijuana had a much higher incidence of fatal opioid overdoses.* The authors made sure to note that neither the earlier nor the latter study provides evidence of a causal

States Legalizing Medical Marijuana Showed an Increase in Opioid Abuse

- Bachuber study (2014)
  1999 to 2010: 21% drop in fatal opioid deaths

- Stanford study (2019)
  1999 to 2017: 23% increase in fatal opioid deaths

relationship between marijuana access and opioid overdose deaths.

They concluded the article with this quote: "Research into the therapeutic potential of cannabis should continue, but the claim that enacting medical cannabis laws will reduce opioid overdose death should be met with skepticism."

"If you think opening a bunch of dispensaries is going to reduce opioid deaths, you'll be disappointed. We don't think cannabis is killing people, but we don't think it's saving people," said Keith Humphreys, the author of the study who is a professor of psychiatry and behavioral sciences at Stanford University.

Trying to substitute cannabis use for opioid use has ended up, like so many others, being another promising benefit of marijuana that hasn't come to fruition.

KEY POINTS

The research data is unequivocal: medical marijuana is not a solution to the opioid epidemic. Passing medical marijuana laws has not reduced opioid use, overdoses or deaths. In fact, the most recent research seems to suggest that states which passed medical marijuana laws have experienced an increase in opioid deaths, but these studies did not prove causation. Finally, studies suggest that people who use marijuana are at an increased risk for using and misusing opioids.

CITATIONS

1   Bachhuber M et al., "Medical Cannabis Laws and Opioid Analgesic Overdose Mortality in the United States, 1999–2010," *JAMA Intern Med* 2014; 174(10):1668–1673.
2   Olfson M, Wall M, et al., "Cannabis Use and Risk of Prescription Opioid Use Disorder in the United States," *American Journal of Psychiatry* 2018; 175(1):47-53.
3   Campbell G et al., "Effect of cannabis use in people with chronic non-cancer pain pre-

scribed opioids: findings from a 4-year prospective cohort study," *Lancet Public Health* 2018; 3(7):341-350.

4   Caputi T et al., "Medical Marijuana Users are More Likely to Use Prescription Drugs Medically and Nonmedically," *Journal of Addiction Medicine* 2018; 12(4): 295–299.

5   Humphreys K et al., "Should Physicians Recommend Replacing Opioids with Cannabis?" *JAMA* 2019; 321(7):639-640.

6   Shover at al., "Association between medical cannabis laws and opioid overdose mortality has reversed over time" *Proceedings of the National Academy of Science* 2019; 116(26): 12624-12626.

CHAPTER 19

Myth #5: No One Has Ever Died from Marijuana

"It looked like it was all THC because her autopsy showed no physical disease or afflictions that were the cause of death. There was nothing else identified in the toxicology—no other drugs, no alcohol. There was nothing else."
—Christy Montegut, MD, Coroner

When we evaluate intoxicant substances that can cause death, marijuana is one of the least likely drugs to cause a fatal overdose. However, it is still toxic when the dose is large enough, and it can lead to premature deaths indirectly.

Not a day goes by that I do not see some post on social media claiming there has never been a death due to marijuana. It simply isn't true. Spreading this fairy tale is dangerous because it plays into the myth of marijuana as a completely natural and entirely safe way to get high. Let's look at the facts.

DIRECT FATAL OVERDOSES FROM MARIJUANA ARE RARE

It would take more than 500 times the dose in one marijuana cigarette to receive a fatal dose of THC. This is in sharp contrast to opioids where the lethal dose is close to the dose needed to get high.

However, the Centers for Disease Control and Prevention (CDC) has been quietly reporting a very small number of deaths solely from marijuana—typically fewer than 20 deaths per year—in its WONDER database for years. There is a good reason for the low number of fatal deaths. Cannabinoid receptors, unlike opioid receptors, are *not* located in the brainstem. The brainstem can be thought of as the master control center for vital body functions, including breathing, swallowing, heart rate and blood pressure. These functions tend to be unaffected by cannabinoids unless given in very high doses, which is in sharp contrast to opioids.

LETHAL DOSING

While the lethal dose (LD) of THC has not been well-studied in humans, scientists have estimated the LD50 (see sidebar) by injecting rats with increasingly large doses. As expected, the LD50 for marijuana was hundreds of times the effective dose (ED50), meaning someone would have to take 500 to 1,500 times the normal amount of marijuana in one joint to receive a fatal dose. Alcohol is more dangerous than marijuana when we compare lethal doses. The LD50 for alcohol is 10 drinks all at once, while the effective dose (ED50) is simply one or two drinks. (For heroin, the lethal dose is only five times the effective dose.)

These are population studies, but the LD50 and ED50 for any individual can vary greatly. For instance, the lethal dose of alcohol for any individual depends on how much alcohol a person drinks, the condition of their liver, their overall physical condition, their hydration state, etc., and the same interpersonal variability is true for THC. However, the high LD50/ED50 ratio for THC explains why fatal overdoses are rare.

Lethal Dose (LD50)

LD50 is the dose of a drug required to kill half the members of a tested population after a specified test duration.

Effective Dose (ED50)

ED50 is the dose or amount of drug that produces a therapeutic response or desired effect in some 50% of the subjects.

LD50/ED50 Ratio

The LD50/ED50 ratio is called the Therapeutic Index (TI). If the TI shows a higher value it indicates the greater safety margin of a drug.

VAPING, DRUG MIXING, CARDIOVASCULAR AND SUICIDE DEATHS

Experts have growing concerns that the higher THC concentrations and the new methods of delivery (oils, vaping, dabbing, etc.) could drive us somewhat closer to the fatal overdose level. Vaping is an especially risky behavior.

Christy Montegut, a New Orleans coroner, reported a case in which THC was the only drug in a fatal overdose. According to *Newsweek* on June 7, 2019, the healthy 39-year-old woman was found dead in her apartment after overdosing from vaping THC oil. "It looked like it was all THC because her autopsy showed no physical disease or afflictions that were the cause of death," Montegut explained. "There was nothing else identified in the toxicology—no other drugs, no alcohol. There was nothing else."

It wasn't an isolated case. In the summer of 2019, more than 2,000 people were hospitalized and more than a dozen people died from vaping THC. More than half of the hospitalized patients ended up being admitted to an intensive care unit.[1] CDC Director Robert Redfield responded by stating, "The CDC has been warning about the identified and potential dangers of...vaping since these devices first appeared."

The high LD50/ED50 ratio explains why the fatal drug overdoses from marijuana that do occur often involve risky delivery systems (vaping and dabbing) or drug mixing (marijuana plus something else). Marijuana plus cocaine or marijuana plus heroin is an extremely dangerous and potentially fatal combination. The most frequently encountered substance combination implicated in fatal car accidents is marijuana plus alcohol. Beyond the obvious perils of combining two different intoxicants, alcohol directly increases THC blood levels.

There have been reports of fatal heart attacks, hypertensive episodes and arrhythmias from THC, usually in those with pre-existing cardiac issues.[2,3,4] And, of course, the aspiration of gastric contents into the lung can be fatal with any intoxicant that causes a person to be unconscious.

The risk for suicide attempts has been shown to be elevated seven-fold in regular users of marijuana[5,6] and for completed suicides as high as five-fold.[7]

MARIJUANA CAN KILL IN OTHER WAYS - INDIRECTLY

People will also die as an indirect consequence of taking marijuana. Any drug that impairs physical abilities and cognitive awareness can lead users to place themselves in dangerous and fatal situations.

In March 2014, foreign exchange student Levy Thamba, a 19-year-old college student, traveled to Colorado for spring break to get high. Although unfamiliar with marijuana, he and his friends bought four "Sweet Grass Kitchen" lemon poppy seed cookies (65 mg)—one for each of them. According to the police report, each cookie was listed as a "6.5 Serving" and a cannabis store employee told them to "cut the cookie into six pieces and to only eat one piece at a time." At first, Levy only consumed one-eighth of the cookie. When it did not have an immediate effect, he ate the rest. He then went into a wild THC-induced psychosis, smashing hotel furniture and claiming he was hearing directly from God. Sadly, he ended up jumping off the balcony, falling to his death. The coroner's report cited marijuana intoxication as the cause of death.[8]

Marijuana-related deaths have increased in Colorado as THC was suspected to be the culprit in car accidents, fatal fires, explosions, homicides, accidents and suicides.[9,10,11,12] Fatal stories like this are many but relatively uncommon considering the sheer number of people consuming marijuana. However, a small fraction of a large number can be a large number.

Keep in mind that car accidents, homicides and other accidents can affect others. When one in five users admits to having driven "very high" and more than half (56%) say they have driven within two hours of a dose, everyone on the road is at risk. Cannabis boosts the risk of accidents as much as 14-fold and doubles the odds of a fatal collision.

MARIJUANA CAN KILL SLOWLY

The vast majority of regular marijuana users will not die from a THC overdose, either directly or indirectly. But many will experience a gradual decline in physical, social and emotional health over decades of use, resulting in dysfunctional lives and premature deaths. (See chapters 7 and 15 for a more detailed list of harmful effects.)

When someone has a cannabis use disorder (an addiction), work, school, marriages and relationships tend to suffer, and these can and will cause a poorer quality of life and premature deaths. Of course, there are exceptions to every rule, and I've heard of long-term marijuana users (those clearly with a marijuana use disorder) who seem to have a steady and satisfying life. The same can be said for some alcoholics and heroin addicts, as some people can manage to keep it all together in spite of addiction.

Millions of lives have been ruined and cut short by various intoxicants over the millenniums, and not one intoxicant has ever lived up to its initial hype of being safe. Let's be ready to see a similar scenario play out regarding marijuana.

KEY POINTS

Fatal overdoses from solely THC are rare. However, marijuana has caused and will continue to cause premature untimely deaths. Fatal heart attacks, lung illnesses, car crashes, accidents and suicides have all been related to marijuana use. In addition, many regular users will experience a gradual decline in physical, social and emotional health over decades of use, resulting in dysfunctional lives and premature deaths.

CITATIONS

1   *https://www.msn.com/en-us/news/us/officials-thc-products-linked-to-vaping-related-illnesses/ar-AAHWN83*

2   Mittleman MA et al., "Triggering Myocardial Infarction by Marijuana," *Circulation* 2001;103(23):2805-2809.

3   Thomas G, Kloner RA, Rezkalla S, "Adverse cardiovascular, cerebrovascular, and peripheral vascular effects of marijuana inhalation: what cardiologists need to know," *Am J Cardiol* 2014;113(1):187-190.

4   Jones RT, "Cardiovascular system effects of marijuana," *J Clin Pharmacol* 2002;42(11 Suppl):58S - 63S.

5   Clarke MC, Coughlan H, et al., "The impact of adolescent cannabis use, mood disorder and lack of education on attempted suicide in young adulthood," *World Psychiatry* 2014:13(3):322-323.

6   Sums N, Horwood U, et al., "Young adult sequelae of adolescent cannabis use: an integrative analysis," *Lancet Psychiatry* 2014; 1(4):245-318.

7   Arendt M, Munk-Jorgensen P, et al., "Mortality following treatment for cannabis use disorders: predictors and causes," *J Subst Abuse Treat* 2013; 44(4):400-406.

8   *https://www.denverpost.com/2014/04/17/man-who-plunged-from-denver-balcony-ate-6x-recommended-amount-of-pot-cookie/*

9   Ramaekers JG et al., "Dose related risk of motor vehicle crashes after cannabis use," *Drug Alcohol Depend* 2004;73(2):109-119.

10 Li M-C, Brady JE et al., "Marijuana Use and Motor Vehicle Crashes," *Epidemiol Rev* 2012;34(1):65-72.

11 Asbridge M et al, "Acute cannabis consumption and motor vehicle collision risk: systematic review of observational studies and meta-analysis," *BMJ* 2012;344:e536.

12 Smart Approaches to Marijuana. Lessons Learned from Marijuana Legalization, 2018. *https://learnaboutsam.org/wp-content/uploads/2018/07/SAM-Lessons-Learned-From-Marijuana-Legalization-Digital-1.pdf.*

CHAPTER 20

Myth #6: No One Has Ever Overdosed on Marijuana

"Emergency room records from Dr. Monte's hospital (in Colorado) show a three-fold increase in marijuana cases (overdoses) since the state became the first to allow sales of recreational marijuana in January 2014. Nearly a third of patients were admitted to the hospital, evidence of severe symptoms."
—CBS News (March 26, 2019)[1]

E very day in just about every emergency room in our country, an emergency room physician will attend to a patient suffering from a THC overdose or poisoning. Yet, internet and social media sites are overflowing with untrue declarations claiming a person cannot overdose on marijuana.

In a study published in the *Annals of Internal Medicine* (March 2019), researchers reported the results of emergency room records at the UCHealth University of Colorado Hospital, the largest hospital in Colorado. Before the year 2000, emergency rooms hardly ever saw a person with a THC overdose. By 2012, the UCHealth emergency room was seeing an average of one patient every *other* day with a marijuana overdose. By 2016, the count was up to two to three a day. Dr. Andrew Monte, the lead author of the study, anticipates these numbers growing higher with the increased availability of marijuana and the higher THC concentrations, "We may be seeing more adverse drug reactions."[1,2] All of these reports and reviews do not consider marijuana-related accidents and injuries, only marijuana poisonings or overdoses.

These unfortunate people typically present with one of the following overdose symptoms: extreme paranoia, panic attacks, psychotic behaviors, hallucinations, hypotension (low blood pressure), unresponsiveness, vomiting, inability to move, headaches, shortness of breath, heart arrhythmias, dizziness, fall injuries and suicidal ideation.

In this study, 2,567 emergency visits at a Denver hospital were caused by marijuana overdoses from 2012 to 2016. Almost one in five cannabis-related visits (17%) was for uncontrolled bouts of vomiting. One in eight visits (12%) was for acute psychosis, which is when thoughts and emotions are so impaired that a person without a history of mental disorders loses contact with reality. One of every nine visits (11%) was triggered by edibles. In addition, there has been a disturbing and significant increase in accidental overdoses by infants, children and unwitting adults. Of all the patients seen in the emergency room for marijuana, nearly one-third were seriously ill and needed to be admitted.[1,2,3]

EDIBLES ARE A SPECIAL PROBLEM

Edibles are a particular concern because many people, unaware of the delayed onset (peak levels are one to three hours after ingestion), get impatient for an effect and take more. While edibles make up a small (but rapidly rising) percent of total cannabis sales, they represent a much larger percent of emergency room visits.

In April 2014, Richard Kirk went to a nearby Colorado marijuana store and purchased a "Karma Candy Orange Ginger" treat (100 mg THC) and a "98 Bubba Kush Pre-Roll" joint. He ate part of the candy on the drive back home but saved the joint for a later time. By the time he got home to his wife and three children, he was ranting—apparently in a state of THC-induced psychosis. His wife Kris frantically called 911, but while she was still talking to the 911 dispatcher, he shot her in the head, killing her. Convicted of murder, Mr. Kirk told the judge and the packed courtroom: "I did not know it (marijuana) would affect me the way it did. That's the honest truth, your honor. I know with certainty if I did not ingest that marijuana edible, Kris would still be here today."[4]

In states where marijuana is legal, three disturbing emergency room trends were disclosed in a review published in 2017 in the *American Journal of Health-System*.[3] Please note these reports were published before the 2019 epidemic of vaping illnesses and deaths.

1. **Accidental Pediatric Overdoses:** The review found a significant increase in accidental pediatric overdoses and in the severity of the presenting symptoms.

Emergency room physicians relate this to the high THC concentrations now routinely found in edibles. According to the researchers, "Children are at particular risk of cannabis toxicity because cannabis-containing food products look similar to regular candy." Here is a typical case as related by the physicians:

A 17-month-old boy was brought to the hospital by his parents due to the child's lethargy. They were having difficulty arousing him. When evaluated in the ED, the child was sleepy but responded to painful stimuli. Laboratory test results, a computed tomography (CT) scan of his brain, and lumbar puncture findings were unremarkable. A urine drug screen tested positive for marijuana. After further questioning, the child's father stated that he observed the child eat a chocolate candy 3 hours before the onset of his symptoms. He initially thought it was a regular candy but acknowledged now that it likely contained marijuana.

2. **Cannabis Hyperemesis Syndrome:** This is characterized by persistent and unrelenting vomiting, typically for hours on end. The mechanism for this syndrome is unknown, but is more commonly seen in heavy, regular cannabis users or when occasional users increase their dosage.

3. **Synthetic Cannabinoids Overdoses:** People seeking more intense highs are manufacturing synthetic cannabinoids commonly sold under the names Spice, K2 and Synthetic Marijuana. Crafted to have a higher affinity for cannabinoid receptor sites in the brain than natural cannabis, these chemical analogues give a different, faster and more intense high. Overdoses from synthetic cannabinoids are problematic because of the severity of symptoms and the unknown ingredients. Many of these patients require intensive care unit stays and some have died. Synthetic cannabinoids have been detected in both CBD and THC products.

KEY POINTS

The internet and social media sites are filled with information stating there is no such thing as overdosing on marijuana.

Yet, every day in every emergency room across the country, emergency room physicians tend to patients presenting with marijuana overdoses or THC poisoning. Emergency room visits due to overdoses and accidental consumption have ballooned in areas where marijuana has been legalized.

CITATIONS

1   *https://www.cbsnews.com/news/after-legalization-marijuana-related-er-vis-its-climb-at-colorado-hospital/*

2   Monte AA et al., "Acute Illness Associated with Cannabis Use, by Route of Exposure: An Observational Study," *Ann Intern Med.* 2019;170(8):531-537.

3   Heard K, Marlin M et al., "Common marijuana-related cases encountered in the emergency department," *American Journal of Health-System Pharmacy* 2017;74(22).

4   *https://www.denverpost.com/2017/04/07/richard-kirk-2014-observatory-park-wife-homicide-sentencing/*

CHAPTER 21

Myth #7: Marijuana Can Make a Person More Creative, Mellow and Less Anxious

"The greatest weapon against stress is our ability to choose one thought over another."
—William James, philosopher and psychologist

"I first started smoking weed when I was around 12, and by age 15 I was getting stoned pretty much all day, every day, until one night in my room when I started to develop what I now understand to be psychosis. I could hear people calling for me in my house and would run downstairs to see what was going on, only to see there was no one home. I would hear heavy rainfall on my window, only to look outside and find a still, dry night. It started happening like clockwork: every time I started smoking I would have the same hallucinations. I knew pretty much instantly it was from the weed, but it took a long time to wean myself off it, both because I loved it so much and because it was all my social circle were interested in doing. I stopped smoking fully in my mid-twenties (but started back) when I realized I could get stoned now and again without any of those hallucinations coming back. But now I've pretty much cut it out again because once I start, I can't control myself with it. I'm a stoner at heart, so getting 'a bit' stoned 'now and again' just doesn't do it for me."[1]
—Jo

The upbeat archetype of a marijuana user (as opposed to the "out of touch" user) is of a creative, mellow, less anxious person and someone who is "cool" and would never have a reason to get depressed.

Unfortunately, the studies show this characterization to be another myth. Let's scrutinize each characterization in more detail.

DOES MARIJUANA MAKE PEOPLE MORE CREATIVE?

According to a well-designed and innovative study at Leiden University in the Netherlands, THC only produces an "illusion of enhanced creativity." The researchers were unable to detect any increase in creativity or creative thinking.[2] "The improved creativity that they believe they experience is an illusion," Dr. Lorenza Colzato, assistant professor of neuromodulation of cognition at Institute of Psychology, Leiden University, and one of the authors of the study, said in a statement. "If you want to overcome writer's block or any other creative gap, lighting up a joint isn't the best solution. Smoking several joints one after the other can even be counterproductive to creative thinking."

More recent studies, which delved into the individual elements of creativity, found that THC increased divergent thinking but decreased convergent thinking (see sidebar). Both divergent and convergent thinking are needed for creativity.

Convergent Thinking

Convergent thinking attempts to consider all available information and arrive at the single best possible answer. Most of the thinking called for in schools is convergent, as schools require students to gather and remember information and make logical decisions and answers accordingly.

So, does marijuana make a person creative? At this time, we can safely conclude that using marijuana will hinder the creative process as users will be less able to convert the enhanced "out of the box" thoughts and experiences (divergent thinking) into a tangible creative good (convergent thinking).

DOES MARIJUANA MAKE PEOPLE MORE MELLOW?

THC definitely has a significant subduing and mellowing effect on most people. The distortions of time, sound and space when high are relaxing and will make most users feel less anxious, safe and less stressed. And it is this temporary high state that exemplifies the stereotypic marijuana personality. However, starting in the late 1990s, physicians began seeing more marijuana users with anxiety and panic attacks—the complete opposite of being mellow. Sufferers were experiencing one or more of the following symptoms: a racing heart, severe weakness, dizziness, tingling or numbness in the hands and fingers, terror or impending doom, a fear of passing out, sweats, chest pains, insomnia and shortness of breath. People will readily tell you attacks are one of the most frightening experiences imaginable. Having a panic attack when high on THC is considerably more confusing, terrifying and challenging. Some addiction specialists attribute the increase in panic attacks and anxiety to the higher concentrations of THC and the rising number of regular users.

"The improved creativity that they believe they experience is an illusion...."
—Dr. Lorenza Colzato, assistant professor of neuromodulation of cognition at The Institute of Psychology, Leiden University

Other individuals report experiencing a pleasant and mellow THC high only to be followed by crippling anxiety a couple of hours later. This "anxiety rebound effect" is more common in daily users, can be quite disabling and will often persist for days, weeks and even months after the last joint. Physicians consider this part of the Cannabis Withdrawal Syndrome (CWS). Unfortunately, most people don't know about CWS or the anxiety rebound effect and view another joint as the solution to the anxiety rather than the cause. Well, you can see the problem. Unwitting sufferers will smoke marijuana again to relieve the anxiety and the entire cycle repeats itself becoming more and more severe. Eventually, this may lead to a generalized anxiety disorder, increased daily use and a substance use disorder.[3]

THC AND VIOLENCE

In his book *Tell Your Children: The Truth about Marijuana, Mental Illness and Violence*, Alex Berenson makes persuasive arguments linking marijuana and violence. Researchers have documented for decades that alcohol is a proven risk factor for violence: domestic abuse, assault and even murder. Berenson, an acclaimed former investigative reporter for *The New York Times*, documents that "dozens of studies exist (linking marijuana to violence), covering everything from bullying by high school students to fighting among vacationers in Spain."[4] A 2012 paper in the *Journal of Interpersonal Violence* examined more than 9,000 adolescents and found that marijuana was associated with a doubling of domestic violence.[5]

THC AND DEPRESSION

On the other end of the spectrum are those daily users of marijuana who experience less motivation, decreased appetite, weight loss and lack of energy while also becoming socially withdrawn as they manifest depression-like symptoms. Research has clearly shown that people who use marijuana regularly are more likely to suffer with depression than those who do not, but some have speculated that being depressed leads people to use THC.[6] It's the old "chicken or the egg" question. But clearly, given the strong link with suicide, people predisposed to depression should avoid marijuana.

THC AND PSYCHOSIS

Some users of marijuana will experience frightening hallucinations when high. Some will hear voices, others will see imaginary objects and still others will experience strange "out of body" feelings. Usually, these hallucinations go away on their own with time and rest. But psychiatrists worry these episodes in teens and young adults could be the beginning of a lifelong problem. THC use does increase a person's chance of developing short-term and even long-term psychotic symptoms, like schizophrenia.[4]

"I never used to smoke weed as much as most people my age; for me it was more of a 'once a fortnight' thing to take the edge off of hangovers and comedowns. In 2012, I visited Amsterdam with some seasoned stoners, and on the first day we all went to a cafe and decided to go in on some 'vaporised isolate,' which you inhale from a bag. Sadly, I completely lost it…I lost track of where I was, what was happening, didn't recognize anything around me. To this day, the only way I can describe what happened to me in words is that I got locked inside my own mind. It was like I was thrown all of the world's most challenging philosophical conundrums to deal with all at once, and I couldn't even (tell) my friend what was happening as he walked me around the area to calm me down. I still look back on that holiday and get little flashbacks once every six months or so, which leave me feeling very confused and anxious for about an hour. It's really odd, because I never suffered from anxiety, but for about an hour every six months, I relive the experience—although it's becoming less frequent now. I properly decided to build on life after that, though, and I can honestly say it's helped turn my life into an amazing experience. In a way, I appreciate that it happened."[1]
—Daniel

KEY POINTS

Marijuana will make most users more mellow but less creative. While the effects of THC on personality, anxiety and well-being are very individual, generalized anxiety, panic attacks, depression, hallucinations, violence and even psychosis are becoming increasingly common as regular marijuana use increases and THC levels rise.

CITATIONS

1   *https://www.vice.com/en_uk/article/kbvwez/people-talk-about-the-experience-that-made-them-stop-smoking-weed-weedweek2017*

2   Kowal A et al., "Cannabis and creativity: highly potent cannabis impairs divergent thinking in regular cannabis users," *Psychopharmacology* 2015; 232(6):1123-1134.

3   Hill K, *Marijuana: The Unbiased Truth About the World's Most Popular Weed.* Center City, Minnesota: Hazelden Publishing; 2015.

4   Berenson, Alex, *Tell Your Children: The Truth About Marijuana, Mental Illness, and Violence.* Glencoe, Illinois: Free Press; 2018.

5   Reingle JM, Staras SA, et al., "The Relationship Between Marijuana Use and Intimate Partner Violence in a Nationally Representative, Longitudinal Sample," *Journal of Interpersonal Violence* 2018.

6   National Academies of Science, Engineering and Medicine. The Health Effects of Cannabis and Cannabinoids: The Current State of Evidence and Recommendations for Research. Washington, DC: The National Academies Press; 2017.

CHAPTER 22

Myth #8: Marijuana is Green (Environmentally Friendly)

Marijuana: 1 ounce (indoor) = 280 pounds of CO_2 emissions
Beer: 12-pack = 14 pounds of CO_2 emissions

Although the leaves of the marijuana plant are a beautiful hue of green, cannabis is not an environmentally friendly plant. Marijuana is no longer being primarily grown in small batches by hippie-farmers who love nature and mother earth. Today's marijuana is grown by large commercial agri-corporations with chemists and accountants at their beck and call. Remember, we have not legalized marijuana; instead, we have capitalized, monetized, commercialized and marketed THC.

The outdoor cultivation of marijuana requires land clearing, deforestation, erosion, surface water diversion and the use of polluting pesticides and fertilizers. Indoor cultivation, which increases revenue by shortening the growth cycle, has an even higher environmental cost as it relies heavily on powerful lights, a plentiful water supply and abundant fertilizers.

MARIJUANA IS A THIRSTY PLANT

Compared to hemp and other commercial crops, marijuana requires a comparatively large amount of water. While the average adult human male needs to drink about three liters of water a day, the average mature marijuana plant consumes two to five liters of water daily. In other words, one marijuana plant and one person consume about the same amount of water. When you look over a marijuana field in places like water-challenged California and Colorado, you can see why a discussion about water priorities is urgently needed. Are the benefits of THC to humans worth the negative impact to the environment?[1]

MARIJUANA IS POWER-HUNGRY

In 2012 (long before the recent surge in the marijuana industry), indoor marijuana growers consumed 1% of the nation's electricity, six times the amount of power used by the entire U.S. pharmaceutical industry.[2] "The basic issue is the lighting intensity inside these growing facilities is much, much higher than anything else. They light up these facilities brighter than an operating room," said Ron Flax, the chief building official in Boulder County, Colorado. Another way to look at this is indoor marijuana growing operations consume about $6 billion annually in energy costs, matching the total energy consumption of about 1.7 million American homes.[2] That's significantly more than all the homes in the state of Iowa. Is shortening the growth cycle to increase profit worth the environmental impact?

GREENHOUSE GASES

The pollution of three million cars is equivalent to the annual greenhouse gas pollution from the indoor cannabis industry, estimates Evan Mills, an energy analyst and research affiliate at the University of California at Berkeley. Mills' study, published in *Energy Policy*, also found that for every kilogram of weed produced, an estimated 4.6 kilograms of carbon dioxide is released into the environment.[2] Our question remains the same: are the benefits of THC worth the deleterious effects on the environment?

CONCLUSION

The intent of this chapter is not to nitpick on the marijuana industry. Every industry has challenges with good stewardship of the environment. However, it seems to me that when voters are asked about legalizing marijuana, the environmental impact should at least be discussed and explored.

My neighbors and I recycle extensively, we limit water usage and we are careful to turn off lights. I think we have a moral obligation to ask those promoting the legalization and commercialization of THC in our communities whether marijuana is good for our environment and our planet. Are the benefits of THC to humans worth the harmful effects on the environment?

KEY POINTS

Despite bucolic images of the hippie farmer, today's marijuana is being produced by a sophisticated industrial complex and comes with a significant environmental cost. Marijuana, compared to hemp and other crops, requires a comparatively larger amount of water, fertilizer and pesticide. Indoor cultivation consumes an inordinate amount of electricity and produces excessive greenhouse gases. As a society considering legalization, we need to be asking if the benefits are worth the negative impact on our environment.

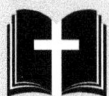

THE CHRISTIAN PERSPECTIVE
CARING FOR THE EARTH

"The earth is the Lord's, and all its fullness, The world and those who dwell therein."
—Psalm 24:1, NKJV

From the beginning, man was given a garden to tend, and every person who has been born since Adam inherits this task. Genesis relates that God gave humans dominion over all the earth with instructions to subdue it. The word "dominion" in this context involves responsibility and accountability—a mandate to care, protect, sustain and enhance the world He lovingly created. Namely, our goal is to use everything our Creator has given us to its greatest good. But the fall caused mankind—that is, all of us—to use creation for selfish purposes. History has taught us that profit and efficiency, when all-consuming, can get in the way of good environmental stewardship. The widespread growth of the marijuana industry, according to scientists, will have a significant impact on the environment due to excessive demands for water, power, pesticides and fertilizers. Managing the environment and caring for the earth is a part of our role as caretakers of this garden we call earth. This requires a thoughtful and circumspect posture in research, prayer and thought.

A PRAYER

Sovereign Lord, You are the creator of the earth. In your wisdom and as a divine blessing, you have allocated to us dominion over the earth's many resources. Forgive us for squandering your treasures in so many ways. Grant us wisdom to use the earth and its resources wisely in the service of people and to the glory of your name. In the name of Jesus, Amen

CITATIONS

1   Carah JK, Howard JK, Thompson SE, et al., "High Time for Conservation: Adding the Environment to the Debate on Marijuana Liberalization," *Bioscience* 2015; 65(8): 822-9.

2   Mills D, The Carbon Footprint of Indoor Cannabis Production," *Energy Policy* 2012; 46: 58-67.

CHAPTER 23

Myth #9: Marijuana is Safe During Pregnancy and When Breastfeeding

"I believe it's beneficial. I don't think it is toxic in any shape or form."
—A pregnant mom when interviewed by a Colorado TV station[1]

Georgette's third pregnancy was the most difficult by far. The only way she could keep food down was by smoking marijuana. A single mom living in Colorado, she was relieved when "the nice lady at the marijuana store" told her marijuana was perfectly safe for morning sickness. "I had two other kids and a demanding job – I wasn't sleeping well – eating poorly – I just needed to survive."

According to an *American Academy of Pediatrics* report (August 2018), marijuana is one of the most widely used substances by pregnant women in the United States and, given the possible medical harms to the unborn baby, this is deeply disconcerting.[2,3] In 2019, U.S. Surgeon General Dr. Jerome Adams stated it clearly and unequivocally, "No amount of marijuana use during pregnancy...is known to be safe."[4] The use of marijuana during pregnancy increased in the state of Washington after legalization[5] and is on the rise nationally.[3]

National and international medical guidelines strongly recommend that pregnant women, and those considering pregnancy, should discontinue all cannabis use.[2,6]

Because of the urgency and seriousness of this problem, physician groups and departments of health have reluctantly invited legal enforcement into the situation. Pregnant women can be subject to child welfare investigations if they have a positive marijuana screen result, even in states where marijuana is legal.[2]

A report in the medical journal *Pediatrics* stated that the legalization of marijuana in some states has given many young women the false impression that it is safe.[2] Aggravating this situation are social media sites and marijuana dispensaries touting the use of marijuana for nausea associated with pregnancy.[1] Unfortunately, women who are breastfeeding are self-medicating with marijuana to ease discomfort and facilitate relaxation.[7]

From 2009 to 2017, cannabis use during the year prior to pregnancy almost doubled, increasing from 7% to 13%.[2,8] In a study conducted in a large hospital system, marijuana use by pregnant women rose by 69% (4.2% to 7.1%) between 2009 and 2016.[8] The statistics are especially grim when we look at pregnant women between the age of 18 and 25: one in every 12 reported using marijuana in the last month.[5] One of every 12 women with mild nausea and vomiting used marijuana and the usage rate increased to one in every nine for those experiencing severe nausea.[5]

THE ENDOCANNABINOID SYSTEM AND FETAL DEVELOPMENT

The research results of Galve-Roperh and his colleagues, experts on the eCB system (see sidebar on next page), demonstrate the "extreme vulnerability" of the developing brain to cannabinoids. A properly functioning endocannabinoid system is essential and crucial for normal fetal brain development, and scientists are worried that delayed or abnormal brain development may be seen in infants exposed to THC *in utero*.

Without going into more detail on this complex scientific system, even a simple understanding of the eCB and its role in the development of the unborn baby should provide a reasonable person with sufficient information to discontinue all marijuana use when pregnant or when considering pregnancy.

THC AND PREGNANCY

THC passes through the placenta and into the circulation of an unborn baby.[5,8] The effects on the unborn are unknown, although there is some evidence that women who use marijuana during pregnancy are more likely to experience placental complications and give birth to babies who are less alert and have lower birth weight. In addition, some early studies are suggesting possible developmental, cognitive issues and heart issues. Studies reported in July 2019 found that 12% of these babies were preterm compared with 6.1% in non-users.[9-14]

A clinically-controlled study published in 2018 found that mothers vulnerable to

Endocannabinoid (eCB) System[22,23]

The endocannabinoid system is a group of endocannabinoids, cannabinoid receptors and enzymes located in the human brain and throughout the entire body.

Studies have revealed that cannabinoids act as regulators for a variety of brain and nervous system processes, including motor learning, appetite, memory, sleep, pain sensation, female reproduction, stress responses and metabolic regulation among other cognitive and physical processes.

We know the eCB plays a role in uterus implantation, is detectable when the human embryo is only one cell and plays a central role in the development of the brain, spinal cord and other organs in infants and children.

mental illness who smoked during pregnancy put their child at higher risk to develop significantly more psychotic symptoms earlier in life compared with mothers who didn't smoke marijuana but had similar vulnerabilities.[15] This study has not been validated by other studies and some have questioned the methodology.

A research letter published in 2019 in *JAMA Psychiatry* found that there was a small increase in psychosis during middle childhood when unborn children were exposed to marijuana. Prenatal cannabis exposure after, but not before, maternal knowledge of pregnancy increased offspring psychosis risk.[16]

PREGNANCY, DEPRESSION, ANXIETY AND MARIJUANA

I have heard from multiple clinicians that psychiatrists and obstetricians have reported that some pregnant women on medications for depression and/or anxiety are replacing them with marijuana because "it's safer, natural and green." According to a medical study, nearly 70% of Colorado dispensaries recommended the treatment of medical marijuana during pregnancy.[15] In that study, researchers called dispensaries, told them they were pregnant and recorded the phone conversations. In one case, a dispensary employee was recorded telling a pregnant mom, "Edibles wouldn't hurt the (unborn) child, they'd be going through your (digestive) tract."[17]

MARIJUANA AND BREASTFEEDING

In a study of 50 breastfeeding women who used marijuana, THC was detected in nearly two-thirds of breast milk samples and up to six days after the last marijuana use.[18] In daily users, THC can accumulate in human breast milk, and breast-fed infants will excrete THC in their urine for weeks depending on the exposure.

Sedation and reduced muscle tone have been observed in infants exposed to THC in breast milk. Evidence seems to also show that exposure to THC in the first month of life could result in decreased motor development at one year of age and perhaps beyond. Because a baby's brain is still forming, experts worry that THC consumed in breast milk could affect brain development into childhood and possibly adulthood, but long-term studies have not been done and won't be known for decades.[2,19,20]

The recommendations are clear: women who are contemplating pregnancy, are pregnant or are breastfeeding should not use marijuana. Pregnant mothers suffering with severe nausea and vomiting should reach out to their obstetrician for more effective and safer treatments. Parents of children should be aware of the dangers of passive smoke and refrain from using marijuana in the car, home and other enclosed environments. The American College of Obstetricians and Gynecologists have stated emphatically that "women who are pregnant or contemplating pregnancy should be encouraged to discontinue marijuana use. Women reporting marijuana use should be counseled about concerns regarding potential adverse health consequences of continued use during pregnancy."[21] In 2018, the American Academy of Pediatrics recommended that, "...it is important to advise all adolescents and young women that if they become pregnant, marijuana should not be used during pregnancy."[2]

KEY POINTS

In 2019, U.S. Surgeon General Dr. Jerome Adams stated it clearly, "No amount of marijuana use during pregnancy...is known to be safe." THC passes into unborn babies and into breast milk. Studies suggest that early exposure to marijuana can adversely affect both the placenta and the unborn baby.

Delayed or abnormal brain development is the main concern. In addition, women who use marijuana during pregnancy are more likely to experience placental complications and give birth to babies who are less alert, have lower birth weight and have possible heart issues. The long-term effects of marijuana on the unborn baby are unknown and won't be known for decades, but a small increase in psychosis has been seen in middle childhood.

Pregnant women can be subject to child welfare investigations if they have a positive marijuana screen result, even in states where marijuana is legal.

Pregnant mothers suffering with severe morning sickness, anxiety, insomnia or any other symptom should reach out to their obstetrician. There are safer and more effective treatments than marijuana.

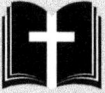

THE CHRISTIAN PERSPECTIVE
PRAYER

Lord Jesus, giver of life,
Every unborn child is tiny, fragile and vulnerable.
Like a little bird in a vicissitudinous sky,
they are subject to winds, storms and dangers.
Please keep them sheltered and out of harm's way.

Grant every mother rest, peace, hope and love
when anxious fears come,
when fatigue and concerns threaten to overwhelm.
Guide every mother to make good choices
despite the stresses of life and worries of pregnancy.

Grant each child a full term of nurture,
a life full of faith and hope.
Please keep watch over the mother and baby,
may they grow together in love.
Give each child parents who cherish and protect,
teach and guide.

I pray for grace and peace for every mother and father
may they accept God's will in all things.
In the name of Jesus.
Amen

CITATIONS

1   *https://denver.cbslocal.com/2016/07/11/marijuana-pregnant-thc-positive-babies-colorado/*

2   Ryan S, et al., "Marijuana Use During Pregnancy and Breastfeeding: Implications for Neonatal and Childhood Outcomes," *Pediatrics* 2018; 142(3): 1-15.

3   Results from the 2018 National Survey on Drug Use and Health: Detailed Tables, SAMHSA, CBHSQ. Accessed on 09/01/19 on *https://www.samhsa.gov/data/sites/default/files/cbhsq-reports/NSDUHDetailedTabs2018R2/NSDUHDetTabsSect1pe2018.htm*

4   *https://www.hhs.gov/surgeongeneral/reports-and-publications/addiction-and-substance-misuse/advisory-on-marijuana-use-and-developing-brain/index.html*

5   Grant TM, Graham JC, Carlini BH, Ernst CC, Brown NN., "Use of marijuana and

other substances among pregnant and parenting women with substance use disorders: Changes in Washington state after marijuana legalization," *Journal of Studies on Alcohol and Drugs* 2018; 79(1):88-95.

6   American College of Obstetricians and Gynecologists. Marijuana Use During Pregnancy and Lactation. (2017). Retrieved from *https://www.acog.org/Clinical-Guidance-and-Publications/Committee-Opinions/Committee-on-Obstetric-Practice/Marijuana-Use-During-Pregnancy-and-Lactation*

7   Adashi EY, "Brief Commentary: Marijuana Use During Gestation and Lactation— Harmful Until Proved Safe Marijuana Use During Gestation and Lactation," *Annals of Internal Medicine* 2019; 170(2): 122.

8   Brown et al., "Trends in Marijuana Use Among Pregnant and Non-Pregnant Reproductive-Aged Woman," *JAMA* 2017; 317(2) 207 – 209.

9   Volkow N et al., "Self-reported Medical and Nonmedical Cannabis Use Among Pregnant Women in the United States," *JAMA* 2019;322(2):167-169.

10   Fried, PA, Watkinson, B and Gray, R., "Differential effects on cognitive functioning in 9-to 12-year-olds prenatally exposed to cigarettes and marihuana," *Neurotoxicol Teratol* 1998;20(3): p. 293-306.

11   Leech, SL, et al., "Prenatal substance exposure: effects on attention and impulsivity of 6-year-olds," *Neurotoxicol Teratol* 1999; 21(2):109-18.

12   Goldschmidt, L, et al., "Prenatal marijuana exposure and intelligence test performance at age 6," *J Am Acad Child Adolesc Psychiatry* 2008 47(3):254-63.

13   Campolongo P, et al., "Developmental consequences of perinatal cannabis exposure: behavioral and neuroendocrine effects in adult rodents," *Psychopharmacology* 2011; 214:5–15.

14   Warner, TD et al., "It's not your mother's marijuana: effects on maternal-fetal health and the developing child," *Clin Perinatology* 2014; 41(4):877-94.

15   Bolhuis K, Kushner SA, et al., "Maternal and paternal cannabis use during pregnancy and the risk of psychotic-like experiences in the offspring," *Schizophrenia Research* 2018; 202:322-327.

16   Fine JD, Moreau AL et al., "Association of Prenatal Cannabis Exposure with Psychosis Proneness Among Children in the Adolescent Brain Cognitive Development (ABCD) Study," *JAMA Psychiatry* 2019; 76(7):762-764.

17   Dickson, B et al., "Recommendations From Cannabis Dispensaries About First-Trimester Cannabis Use," *Obstetrics & Gynecology* 2018; 131(6) 1031-1038.

18   Perez-Reyes M et al., "Presence of Δ9-tetrahydrocannabinol in human milk," N Engl J Med 1982; 307: p. 819–20.

19   Garry A et al., "Cannabis and breastfeeding". *J Toxicol* 2009;2009:596149.

20   Larson JJ et al., "Cognitive and Behavioral Impact on Children Exposed to Opioids During Pregnancy," *Pediatrics* 2019; 144 (2).

21   American College of Obstetricians and Gynecologists: Marijuana use during pregnancy and lactation. Committee Opinion No.722. *Obstet Gynecol* 2017;130(4):e205-e209.

22   Galve-Roperh I, Palazuelos J, Aguado T, Guzman M. The endocannabinoid system and the regulation of neural development: potential implications in psychiatric disorders. *Eur Arch Psychiatry Clin Neurosci.* 2009;259:371–82.

23   Maccarrone M, Valensise H, Bari M, Lazzarin N, Romanini C, Finazzi-Agrò A (2000). "Relation between decreased anandamide hydrolase concentrations in human lymphocytes and miscarriage". *Lancet.* 355 (9212): 1326–9

CHAPTER 24

Myth #10: We Can Limit Marijuana Use to Adults and Keep It Away from Young People

"I don't do it (marijuana) anymore. Why? The truth is I don't really want to set a (bad) example to my kids and grandkids. It's now a parent thing."
—Paul McCartney, musician[1]

"I know you're supposed to tell kids not to do drugs, but, kids, do it! Do weed! Don't do the other stuff, but weed is good!"
—Kevin Smith, Filmmaker, actor

Our history with cigarettes, alcohol and prescription drugs, as well as our experience in states where marijuana has already been legalized, tells us emphatically that an increase in overall accessibility and availability increases teen usage. It is beyond the bounds of possibility and contrary to reason to think we can limit marijuana to adults only.

Everyone, even ardent cannabis enthusiasts, agrees that, as a society, we need to protect our young people from today's high potency marijuana. Well, almost everyone.

TEEN-DIRECTED MARKETING

One of the most outrageous aspects of the legalization of marijuana has been the blatant marketing to young people.[1] Manufacturers and marijuana business owners know it is in their best interest to get people using marijuana when they are young, as a certain percentage will become customers for life. If this sounds too draconian or conspiratorial to you, just look at the playbook from Big Tobacco and Big Alcohol from the 1950s through the early 2000s.

Federal district judge Gladys Kessler clearly outlined tobacco company intent, strategies and disregard for the human tragedy and social costs in a 2006 ruling: "Defendants (tobacco companies) have known many of these (medical) facts for at least 50 years or more. Despite that knowledge, they have consistently, repeatedly, and with enormous skill and sophistication, denied these facts to the public, to the Government, and to the public health community. Moreover, in order to sustain the economic viability of their companies, Defendants have denied that they marketed and advertised their products to children under the age of eighteen and to young people between the ages of eighteen and twenty-one in order to ensure an adequate supply of 'replacement smokers,' as older ones fall by the wayside through death, illness, or cessation of smoking. In short, Defendants have marketed and sold their lethal product with zeal, with deception, with a single-minded focus on their financial success, and without regard for the human tragedy or social costs that success exacted."[2]

Big Alcohol has historically reached out to teens and college students through specific and targeted marketing and advertising methods. And the reasons are all too clear. Even though drinking alcohol by persons under the age of 21 is illegal, people aged 12 to 20 years drink 11% of all the alcohol consumed in the United States, according to the Centers for Disease Control and Prevention (CDC).

According to a September 2019 article in the medical journal *Addictive Behaviors*, young adults were almost twice as likely as older adults to start vaping because of the kid-friendly flavors.[3,4] Marijuana cookies, candies, sodas, gummy bears, gum, breath mints, etc. are all teen-friendly products, and manufacturers know it. Just like with tobacco and alcohol, there is enormous skill and sophistication in their strategies.

MARIJUANA USE IN TEENS HAS BEEN NORMALIZED

Despite the known risks, high school students' perception of the harm from regular marijuana use has been steadily declining over the last decade.[5] The movement to legalize marijuana, supportive politicians, celebrity endorsements, influential marketing groups and social media has had a disproportionately large impact on the attitudes of young people. Our culture has normalized marijuana use to such a degree that teens and college students who don't use marijuana report feeling marginalized and isolated.

From the Surgeon General's Report (August 2019)

"Frequent marijuana use during adolescence is associated with changes in the area of the brain involved with attention, memory, decision-making, and motivation. Deficits in attention and memory have been detected in marijuana-using teens even after a month of abstinence. Marijuana can also impair learning in adolescents. Chronic use is linked to declines in IQ, school performance that jeopardizes professional and social achievement, and life satisfaction. Regular use of marijuana in adolescence is linked to increased rates of school absence and drop-out as well as suicide attempts.

Marijuana use increases the risk for psychotic disorders, such as schizophrenia. This risk increases with the frequency of use, potency of the marijuana product, and as the age at first use decreases. Adolescent marijuana is often linked with other substance use. In 2017, teens 12-17 reporting frequent use of marijuana showed a 130% greater likelihood of misusing opioids. Marijuana's increasingly widespread availability in multiple and highly potent forms, coupled with a false and dangerous perception of safety among youth, merits a nationwide call to action."[6]

"NO AMOUNT OF MARIJUANA USE DURING ADOLESCENCE IS KNOWN TO BE SAFE"

U.S. Surgeon General Dr. Jerome Adams has stated it unequivocally and emphatically, "No amount of marijuana use during...adolescence is known to be safe."[6] The American Academy of Child and Adolescent Psychiatry (May 2017) has staunchly opposed the legalization of marijuana and, in their position paper, they state their reasons clearly:

1. The legalization of marijuana will "decrease adolescent perception of marijuana's harmful effects."

2. The legalization of marijuana will "increase marijuana use among parents and caretakers, and increase adolescent access to marijuana, all of which reliably predict increased rates of adolescent marijuana use and associated problems."

3. The legalization of marijuana has "immediate and long-term implications" including "marijuana's deleterious effects on adolescent cognition, behavior, and brain development."

4. The legalization of marijuana will increase the "risk of motor vehicle acci-

dents, sexual victimization, academic failure, lasting decline in intelligence measures, psychological and occupational impairment."[20]

LEGALIZATION INCREASES TEEN AND YOUNG ADULT USE

Surely our experience with cigarettes, alcohol and prescription drugs should persuade us that increasing overall accessibility and availability boosts teen usage. This truth is already manifesting itself in states where medical and recreational marijuana have been legalized:

- Since Colorado, Washington, Oregon, Alaska and the District of Columbia legalized marijuana, past-month use of marijuana has continued to rise above the national average among youths aged 12 to 17 in all five jurisdictions.[7,8]

- Alaska and Oregon are leading the nation in past-year marijuana use among youths aged 12 to 17.[7]

- Colorado currently holds the top ranking for first-time marijuana use among youths, representing a 65% increase in the years since legalization.[8]

- Young adult use (youth aged 18 to 25) in legalized states is increasing.[7]

- Colorado toxicology reports show the percentage of adolescent suicide victims testing positive for marijuana has increased.[8]

- In Anchorage, Alaska, school suspensions for marijuana use and possession increased more than 141% from 2015 (when legalization was implemented) to 2017.[9]

- A study in Colorado found that about 50% of youths in outpatient substance abuse treatment reported using diverted marijuana.[10] ("Diverted marijuana" is medical marijuana given to someone for a medical condition but the patient turns around and sells it to another for profit. This is not an uncommon occurrence.)

MARIJUANA AND THE DEVELOPING BRAIN

Medical science has clearly shown that cannabis has many more negative effects on teens and young adults when compared with adult use.[11,12] THC binds to cannabinoid receptors involved with thinking, decision-making, memory, pleasure, coordination, appetite and time perception. These cannabinoid receptors are critical for brain development, particularly the formation of brain circuits important for decision-making, complex thinking and responding to stress.

The medical studies are clear: regular marijuana use hinders frontal-executive brain function. This effect is particularly pernicious and persistent in teens. There is concern by addiction psychiatrists that regular marijuana use will have long-lasting effects on brain development in young people. For instance, teens who began smoking marijuana regularly (more than four times per week) before the age of 16 performed poorly on neurocognitive tests—including IQ tests—compared with non-users.[6,13,14] Stopping marijuana use for periods of more than a year did not result in IQ levels returning to normal, worrying physicians that the damage could be permanent. A recent study showed that even occasional marijuana use was linked with changes in the size of key brain structures.[14]

MARIJUANA AFFECTS TEENS SOCIALLY

The regular use of marijuana in teens increases risky behaviors, concentration problems and poor performance in school. In addition, THC in teens has been associated with increased risk of developing schizophrenia, other psychoses, anxiety problems and depression.[13]

> "I'm the medical director of an adolescent substance abuse program, and we noticed in 2009 at the beginning of the year that we were not very busy, and at the end of the year we ended up having probably tripled our referrals to the adolescent substance abuse treatment program. And 95 percent of our referrals are for marijuana."
> —Dr. Christian Thurstone, Past President of the Colorado Child and Adolescent Psychiatric Society[20]

MARIJUANA AS A GATEWAY TO ADDICTION AND HARDER DRUGS IN TEENS

You don't hear much about marijuana as a gateway drug to harder drugs, and that is because studies suggest it is not as significant an issue in adults. Teens with a marijuana use disorder, however, are more likely to progress to more dangerous drugs.[13,15]

The use of nicotine, alcohol or cannabis is almost always seen before the use of other drugs.[14] Animal studies have been helpful in understanding how THC affects the brain. In one study, rodents were repetitively given THC when young, and they were more likely to show addiction-like behaviors. Interestingly, they also exhibited a heightened response to other addictive substances—like opioids and nicotine—in the "reward" areas of the brain.[16,17] These findings support the theory of marijuana being a gateway drug. Fortunately, the vast majority of people who use marijuana will not go on to use other drugs.

UNINTENTIONAL INGESTIONS BY CHILDREN

The pediatric medical literature has documented a significant increase in unintentional marijuana ingestions by young children over the last few years.[21,22] The most recent review of reports to poison control centers,[23] found a significant increase in unintentional pediatric marijuana ingestions that was temporally and geographically associated with the legalization of marijuana.[18]

Between 2009 and 2017, the annual unintentional ingestions (those reported to poison control centers) have increased every year by an average of 27%. Almost three of every four marijuana poisonings occurred in children aged two years or younger. More than 2% of these children exhibited life-threatening symptoms or significant disability, and almost 1% required intubation. Dr. Lauren Westafer said this "trend calls attention to the potential public health consequences of legalized marijuana for a vulnerable population."[18]

PASSIVE MARIJUANA SMOKE

In 2018, researchers investigated trends in cannabis use among parents with children at home from 2002 to 2015. Past-month cannabis use among parents with children at home increased from 4.9% in 2002 to 6.8% in 2015. The researchers cited data suggesting that cannabis smoke "carries health risks similar to, or worse than" secondhand tobacco smoke. They concluded with the statement that parents need "education about protecting children from marijuana products, paraphernalia, waste and smoke."[19]

KEY POINTS

Our history with cigarettes, alcohol and prescription drugs, as well as our experience in states where marijuana has already been legalized, tells us emphatically that an increase in overall accessibility and availability increases teen use of marijuana. It is beyond the bounds of possibility and contrary to reason to think we can limit marijuana to adults only.

U.S. Surgeon General Dr. Jerome Adams said, "No amount of marijuana use during…adolescence is known to be safe." The legalization of marijuana has given teens a false sense of safety. This is disturbing because marijuana use in teens has many more negative effects when compared with adult use: increased addiction rates, deleterious effects on brain development, increased risk of developing schizophrenia and psychosis, loss of concentration, poor performance in school and athletics, declines in IQ scores and an increase in risky behaviors.

People who begin using marijuana before the age of 18 are four to seven times more likely to develop a marijuana use disorder (addiction) than adults and are more likely to advance to harder drugs. Any drug use by a young person should be a cause for concern.

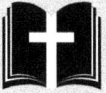

THE CHRISTIAN PERSPECTIVE
IS IT WRONG OR RIGHT?

"What's wrong?" asked the concerned mom to her 17-year-old daughter. "Did anything bad happen at youth group?"

"Oh nothing."

"Then, why are you so quiet and disturbed?" The two were close and moms have a way....

"Well...after youth group, Mom, we all went to the park...it was great fun. But soon, Karen's older brother, Tom, came by with some friends and started smoking pot, I mean marijuana. They asked me if I wanted some. Karen and others laughingly agreed but I didn't...at first. It seemed like a lot of fun so eventually I tried it also."

Mom's face dropped noticeably. "You did?" She immediately regretted her harsh and shrill tone and added meekly, "But I'm glad you told me."

"I'm sorry, Mom. But it is legal. Tom is 20 and next year it is legal for me. I mean...nicotine is a drug, so is caffeine and alcohol. Right? Even TV is addictive, and you watch it a lot. And the Bible never speaks out against marijuana."

This fictitious account highlights that marijuana will become much more available to teens in upcoming years, especially in states where it is legalized. It also illustrates the importance for churches, youth groups and parents to know the facts about marijuana. Since the Bible doesn't address marijuana specifically, one of the most important things we can do is move our teens and young people away from the "Is it wrong or right?" question to the "Is it wise?" question. We discussed the necessity of this paradigm shift in the Christian Perspective section of chapter 10. I suggest you review this in detail as this concept is especially important for teens.

A PRAYER

Father of all, I pray for all the children. Forgive our failings as their mothers and fathers. I pray they would see you as their Father, deliverer and strength. Would you be their counselor? May you and you alone be their salvation, helper and healer. May their character and heart be bigger than their talent and income. Would you be their treasure? I pray their hearts would break when others suffer and they would be compelled to action on their behalf. I pray hardship and temptation would teach them to depend on you and no one else. May your Holy Spirit protect their bodies, guard their minds and center their souls until their journey on this orb is over.
In the name of Jesus, Amen

CITATIONS

1   *https://www.independent.co.uk/news/people/paul-mccartney-quit-cannabis-because-he-didnt-want-to-set-a-bad-example-to-his-grandchildren-10286647.html*

2   *https://www.wilx.com/content/news/Big-Tobacco-forced-to-admit-the-truth-about-dangers-of-smoking-460252283.html*

3   Landry LL, Groom AL et al., "The role of flavors in vaping initiation and satisfaction among U.S. adults," *Addiction Behaviors* 2019;99.

4   *https://newsroom.heart.org/news/study-finds-flavors-play-a-role-in-initiation-addiction-to-e-cigarette-use?preview=9115*

5   Johnston LD et al., "Monitoring the future national survey results on drug use, 1975 – 2018: Overview, key findings on adolescent drug use," Ann Arbor: Institute for Social Research, The University of Michigan.

6   *https://www.hhs.gov/surgeongeneral/reports-and-publications/addiction-and-substance-misuse/advisory-on-marijuana-use-and-developing-brain/index.html*

7   Results from the 2018 National Survey on Drug Use and Health: Detailed Tables, SAMHSA, CBHSQ. Accessed on 09/01/19 on *https://www.samhsa.gov/data/sites/default/files/cbhsq-reports/NSDUHDetailedTabs2018R2/NSDUHDetTabsSect1pe2018.htm*

8   Colorado Department of Public Health & Environment. (2016). As reported in Monitoring Health Concerns Related to Marijuana in Colorado.

9   Wohlforth, C. (2018, January 11). Marijuana school suspensions more than doubled after legalization. *Anchorage Daily News.*

10 Wilkinson ST et al., "Marijuana legalization: Impact on physicians and public health," *Annual Review of Medicine* 2016, 67, 453–466.

11 Lisdahl KM et al., "Dare to delay? The impacts of adolescent alcohol and marijuana use onset on cognition, brain structure, and function," *Front Psychiatry* 2013;4:53.

12 Silins E, Horwood LJ, Patton GC, et al., "Young adult sequelae of adolescent cannabis use: an integrative analysis," *Lancet Psychiatry* 2014;1(4):286-293.

13 National Academies of Science, Engineering and Medicine. The Health Effects of Cannabis and Cannabinoids: The Current State of Evidence and Recommendations for Research. Washington, DC: The National Academies Press; 2017.

14 *https://www.sciencedaily.com/releases/2014/08/140809141436.htm*

15 Secades-Villa, R., Garcia-Rodríguez, O., Jin C.J., Wang, S., & Blanco, C., "Probability and predictors of the cannabis gateway effect: A national study." *International Journal of Drug Policy* 2015, 26(2), 135–142.

16 Panlilio LV, Zanettini C, Barnes C et al., "Prior exposure to THC increases the addictive effects of nicotine in rats," *Neuropsychopharmacol* 2013;38(7):1198-1208.

17 Cadoni C et al., "Behavioural sensitization after repeated exposure to Delta 9-tetrahydrocannabinol and cross-sensitization with morphine," *Psychopharmacology* 2001;158(3):259-266.

18 *https://www.jwatch.org/na49236/2019/06/03/unintentional-marijuana-ingestions-young-children*

19 Goodwin RD et al., "Trends in Cannabis and Cigarette Use Among Parents with Children at Home: 2002 to 2015," *Pediatrics* 2018; 141(6).

20 *https://www.aacap.org/AACAP/Policy_Statements/2014/aacap_marijuana_legalization_*

policy.aspx

21 *JAMA Pediatrics* 2016; 170:e160971

22 *J Emerg Med* 2019; 56:398

23 *Pediatr Emerg Care* 2019 May 1

24 Maccarrone M, Valensise H, Bari M, Lazzarin N, Romanini C, Finazzi-Agrò A (2000). "Relation between decreased anandamide hydrolase concentrations in human lymphocytes and miscarriage". *Lancet.* 355 (9212): 1326–9

CHAPTER 25

Conclusion: The American Dream

"I don't care what people say about marijuana or how bad they say it is for my lungs, my liver, or my brain—I'm going to have my bong next to my bed on the day I die. It will be the last thing I look at when I leave this earth."
— Emily, 15 years old

I love going to the beach and body-surfing the waves. When my kids were young, I always warned them about the second wave. The first wave knocks you silly, making you less aware of the arrival of the second wave.

The first wave was the opioid epidemic. More Americans died from drug overdoses this year than during the entirety of the Vietnam War.[1] My research on this book has convinced me that a second and more insidious wave is coming—it's the marijuana wave. Marijuana's risks are different from opioids, but they are no less real.

Our current situation in the United States is the worst of all worlds. Marijuana has become dangerously potent. It is legal in some states and illegal in others. A widespread decrease in the public's perception of risk has flooded the nation. Usage by teens and young people is rising, and the daily consumption by adults continues to grow.

In this book, I've expressed my reasons and recommendations regarding medical marijuana, recreational marijuana and the decriminalization of marijuana. On this journey, we have come to appreciate the rigors and beauty of the FDA process for regulating medications; plus, we are now familiar with the three marijuana-derived prescription medications that have already helped tens of thousands of people. We are optimistic about ongoing research, and we are hopeful the many potential medical benefits from cannabinoids will be realized in our lifetime.

But we have also learned the dangers cannabis poses to adolescents, pregnant women, people predisposed to mental illness, the elderly and society. We have seen how profit, politics and personal freedom assertions have prevailed over medical science, thereby subjecting millions to fraudulent health claims and dangerous self-treatment. We have learned firsthand the dangers of capitalizing and commercializing an addictive and potentially dangerous substance. We continue to grapple with a difficult policy dilemma: how do we reduce unnecessary, excessive and expensive arrests and eliminate racial disparities in enforcement, while also not increasing marijuana use, accessibility and addictions?

> "In the United States the difficulties are not a Minotaur or a dragon—not imprisonment, hard labor, death, government harassment, and censorship—but cupidity, boredom, sloppiness, indifference. Not the acts of a mighty, all-pervading, repressive government but the failure of a listless public to make use of the freedom that is its birthright."
> —Aleksandr Solzhenitsyn, Harvard Commencement Address, 1978

This book started out as a book about marijuana, but my focus changed about halfway through the process. For me, questions about marijuana ended up becoming questions about the American dream. What kind of a country do we want 50 years from now?

Is the American dream about personal freedoms so expansive that we are free to harm our children, friends and neighbors in the search for profit, personal freedom and tax dollars? Does the American concept of freedom comprise enough self-discipline that we stand united to protect our young people from pernicious and addictive substances that will have short-term and long-term effects on their bodies and brains? Is part of the American dream the large-scale commercialization, capitalization and marketing of an addictive substance?

Does marijuana increase our capacity for relational connection? Does THC increase our sense of purpose and love of neighbor? Does cannabis increase human dignity? Does THC make our neighborhoods better, our marriages stronger, our streets safer, our children healthier?

Or is it more likely to lead to a penurious life and an impoverished nation? Do we

What's Become of Becoming?

"The question to be asked at the end of an educational step is not 'What has the student learned? but what has the student become?'"
—President James Monroe

want to be a nation where people are always seeking another drug high? Have we forgotten the lesson of China and how it toppled under the weight of addiction?

Sadly and tragically, I believe we have not learned the lessons taught by nicotine, alcohol, opioids and history. I worry the next generation is going to grow up in a country where pervasive marijuana use is accepted and possibly encouraged. I reject the idea that America will be a better country if marijuana is sold on the corner of every Main Street.

But I have hope. I believe the best days for our country can be ahead of us if we commit to being people of good will who are guided by civility and science. I believe people of all stripes will find themselves agreeing on most things about marijuana: we need to protect our young people, keep our roads safe from intoxicated drivers, cultivate a healthy population in body and mind, search for new medications for those suffering, care for our environment, avoid harmful addictions and foster good life habits and practices.

The enemy of civility is contempt for those with different views. By being courteous, merciful and humble, we can and will achieve consensus, agreement and forward movement on creating sensible science-based marijuana policies and laws that promote human flourishing.

Like it or not, the marijuana wave is coming. You will be asked to make substantial and sometimes personal choices regarding marijuana in your home, at your workplace, in your house of worship and at the voting box. Ask yourself: what kind of country do you want 50 years from now?

I hope and pray this book has helped you think more deeply, clearly and honestly about this vitally important issue of our day. And I hope and pray this book has compelled you to action. *Christi vobiscum.*

CITATIONS

1   *https://www.cdc.gov/drugoverdose/index.html*
2   Bennett, A (Editor), *The Valley of Vision*: "The Voyage", Carlisle, Pennsylvania: Banner of Truth Trust Publishing; 1975.

YOYAGE[2]

O Lord of the Oceans,
My little bark sails on a restless sea,
Grant that Jesus may sit at the helm and steer me safely;
Suffer no adverse currents to divert my heavenward course;
Let not my faith be wrecked amid storms and shoals;
Bring me into harbor with flying pennants,
hull unbreached, cargo unspoiled…

The voyage is long, the waves high, the storms pitiless,
but my helm is held steady,
thy Word secures safe passage,
thy grace wafts me onward,
my heaven is guaranteed…

Help me to live circumspectly,
with skill to convert every care into prayer,
Halo my path with gentleness and love…
may I strive to bind up every wound,
and pour oil on all troubled waters.

May the world this day be happier and better because I live.
Let my mast before me be the Savior's cross,
and ever oncoming wave the fountain in his side
Help me, protect me in the moving sea
until I reach the shore of unceasing praise.

Appendices

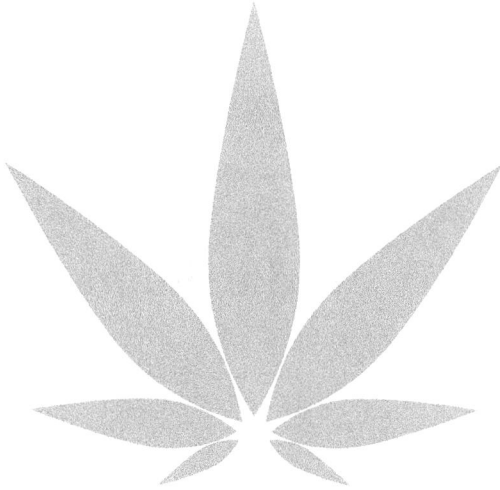

Appendix A
Glossary of Marijuana Terms

Appendix B
CMDA Statement on Medical Marijuana

Appendix C
CMDA Statement on Recreational Marijuana

Acknowledgments

About the Author

Glossary of Marijuana Terms

420

A slang term for the consumption of marijuana. "420-friendly" is a way of saying a place is marijuana friendly. April 20 (4/20) is considered the international day of cannabis pride.

710

710 is OIL flipped upside down and is a slang name for hash oil.

BHO

BHO is an acronym for butane hash oil. It is a highly concentrated and potent form of marijuana made by dissolving the dry flower in a solvent (usually butane). The resulting product has extremely high THC levels (generally more than flowers or hashish) and comes in a consistency of thick, sticky oil. BHO can take different forms, such as honey oil, earwax, crumble, budder or shatter, depending on the manufacturing method.

BLAZE

A slang term for smoking marijuana.

BLUNT

Cannabis wrapped in a tobacco leaf cigar or cigarillo paper. The cigar may be hollowed out and then re-rolled with cannabis. The "blunt" name comes from a popular brand of cigars called "Phillies Blunt." Blunts are thicker than joints and often burn longer.

BONG

A large pipe-like device, usually made of glass, that uses water to diffuse and cool the smoke as you breathe it into your lungs.

BUD

Bud is another name to describe the actual flower of the marijuana plant. These are the fluffy and bulky parts that are harvested. Buds contain the highest concentrations of active cannabinoids.

BUDDER

Another name for marijuana concentrates.

BUDTENDER

This is the employee working behind the counter at the local dispensary or retail cannabis shop.

CANNABINOIDS

Cannabinoids are the naturally occurring compounds unique to the *Cannabis* plant. Marijuana's most well-known cannabinoid is tetrahydrocannabinol (THC) due to the fact that it is the most abundant and also because it produces the psychoactive effects (or the high). CBD is the abbreviation for cannabidiol and is second to THC in terms of the average volume. However, there are more than 100 known cannabinoids, all with varying effects.

Cannabis (CAPITALIZED AND ITALICIZED)

Cannabis is a genus of flowering annual plants in the Cannabaceae family. Botanists would describe *Cannabis* succinctly as an annual herbaceous flowering plant indigenous to Eastern Asia. Within the genus *Cannabis*, there are three main species: *Cannabis sativa*, *Cannabis indica* and *Cannabis ruderalis*. When it is capitalized and italicized, it can refer to hemp or marijuana. *Cannabis ruderalis* is rarely farmed due to its natural lower THC content and small stature.

cannabis (NOT CAPITALIZED OR ITALICIZED)

This is a common name for marijuana.

CBD

CBD is the abbreviation for cannabidiol, one of at least 100 cannabinoids found in cannabis. CBD is second only to THC when it comes to average volume. CBD is not psychoactive. It has the most promise for use as a medical treatment. An FDA-approved medication, Epidiolex, is CBD.

CONCENTRATES

Concentrates are a resinous matrix of high potency cannabinoids (mainly THC) obtained from the cannabis plant by solvent extraction, formed into viscous oil or mass that is similar in appearance to honey or butter. Marijuana enthusiasts will sometimes refer to marijuana concentrates as "710" (that's "OIL" upside down), extract, shatter, wax, honey oil (BHO), budder and taffy.

DAB/DABBING

A dab is a slang term used to refer to a dose of cannabis concentrates "dabbed" onto a red-hot surface (flash-vaporizing) and inhaled. Basically, it is a way to smoke concentrates. The act of "dabbing" refers to partaking in dabs. It is also a slang name for hash oil.

DANK

Dank is a slang word for high-quality cannabis.

DANKRUPT

This means to be out of marijuana.

DISPENSARY

A general term used to refer to a state-sanctioned store that sells marijuana, THC-based products and CBD products. A dispensary may be selling medical marijuana, recreational marijuana or both.

EDIBLES

This is a food or drink containing cannabis. You can infuse virtually anything with cannabis because it is fat-soluble (lipophilic). Cookies, brownies, breads, coffee, drinks, sauces and candies are currently popular edibles.

FLOWERING TIME

Flowering time refers to the time it takes for a plant to produce mature flowers that are ready to harvest. Cannabis flowering times are affected by the length of daily exposure the plant receives to sun.

FLOWER

This is a slang term for marijuana in plant form as opposed to other THC products, or it can simply refer to the flowers of the Cannabis plant.

GANJA

This is a Hindi name for marijuana.

GREENOUT

Greenout is the marijuana equivalent of the alcohol-inspired term "blackout." It describes a level of intoxication so high that one can't remember the events that took place when high.

HASH/HASHISH

Hash is short for hashish. Hashish is a concentrated form of cannabis created by pressing the collected resin from mature flowers into solid blocks. Hash ranges in potency, but it is generally stronger than flowers but weaker than dabs.

HEADSHOP

This is a retail outlet specializing in paraphernalia and items related to cannabis culture.

HEMP

Hemp is a genus of the Cannabis family. It is mainly grown for its stems and stalks, and it can be used in the manufacture of rope, paper, beauty products and a vast array of other products. Hemp has low concentrations of tetrahydrocannabinol (THC), the active psychoactive ingredient in marijuana. The legality of industrial hemp varies widely between countries. In the United States, hemp must have less than 0.3% THC on a dry weight basis. Therefore, hemp has no psychoactive or hallucinogenic properties.

HYBRID

Hybrid refers to a *Cannabis* plant that has been genetically crossed between one or more separate strains of cannabis. Hybrids can happen accidentally or intentionally, but they are usually bred specifically to combine desired traits of the original plants. Most marijuana on the market today is some form of hybrid.

INDICA

Indica is the commonly used name for the *Cannabis indica* species of *Cannabis*. This species tends to be more relaxing and sedating than its cousin, *Cannabis sativa*.

JOINT

A joint is slang for a marijuana cigarette. It is the dried plant rolled in paper and smoked like a cigarette. A "jay" is a shortened version of joint.

KIEF

Kief is now most commonly used as a slang word for marijuana. However, it is the collected amount of trichomes that have been separated from the rest of the marijuana flower. Since trichomes are the sticky crystals that contain the vast majority of the plant's cannabinoids, kief is known to be extremely potent. Hashish is primarily made of kief.

KUSH

Kush is now most commonly used as a slang word for marijuana. However, Kush refers to a line of cannabis plants from the Hindi Kush mountains of Afghanistan, India and Pakistan. Kush strains are *Cannabis indicas* and have a unique and popular aroma.

MARIJUANA

Marijuana is used to define female cannabis plants or their dried flowers. Females are distinct from male plants in that they are the ones that produce flowers which contain the high percentage of cannabinoids that hold both their medicinal and psychoactive properties.

MEDICATING

This is another way of saying, "I'm getting high on THC."

POT

Pot is another slang term for marijuana. It is thought to be a derivative of the Spanish word *potiguaya*.

PRE-ROLL

As the name infers, a pre-roll is a pre-rolled marijuana cigarette, also known as a joint. Many dispensaries have pre-rolls available for sale.

RUDERALIS

Ruderalis is an abbreviation for *Cannabis ruderalis* or *C. ruderalis*. It is a low-THC cannabis variety that is primarily selected by breeders for its CBD-rich genetics. Unlike *Cannabis sativa* and *Cannabis indica*, which use light cycles to flower, ruderalis is an "auto-flowering" variety, meaning it flowers with age. Originating in Russia, ruderalis is a hardy plant that can survive harsh climates.

SATIVA

Sativa is an abbreviation for *Cannabis sativa*. These plants originated outside of the Middle East and Asia but are also common in areas such as South America, the Caribbean, Africa and Thailand. These strains tend to grow taller (usually over five feet) and take longer to flower. When consumed, *C. sativa* plants tend to produce more hallucinogenic and stimulating effects when compared to its cousin *C. indica*.

SHATTER

Shatter is a term used to refer to the purest form of a BHO extract. It is brittle, usually transparent and can break like glass.

STRAIN

A strain is a very specific variety of plant species. Strains are developed to produce distinct desired traits in the plant and are usually named by their breeders. Because there are more than 100 different cannabinoids, producers can develop an infinite number of different combinations or strains.

THC

THC is an abbreviation for delta 9-tetrahydrocannabinol. It is the most prevalent and available cannabinoid in marijuana plants. THC is also the component in marijuana that is responsible for the psychoactive effects or the high. It serves as a natural defense for the plant against pests.

TINCTURE

A tincture is an alcohol-extracted liquid cannabis extract. Tinctures are usually placed under the tongue with a dropper, where they are absorbed quickly. Effects can be felt within minutes. Tinctures can also be mixed into a drink, but the effects will take longer because the tinctures will be absorbed by the digestive system.

TOP SHELF

This is a slang word to refer to high concentration THC.

TRICHOMES

Trichomes are the resin-producing glands of the Cannabis plant. They contain the highest concentrations of THC, CBD and all of the "minor" cannabinoids.

VAPORIZER (VAPING)

A vaporizer is a hand-held device used to consume marijuana. It heats either flowers or marijuana-infused oils to a temperature that releases a THC-laced vapor. A person then inhales the vapor, not the smoke. Vaporizing produces an effect within minutes (like smoking). In September 2019, the FDA issued a warning because hundreds of people became serious ill, many required mechanical ventilation and some died from vaping THC oil.

WAKE AND BAKE

This means the consumption of cannabis early in the morning.

WAX

Wax is another form of concentrate that has been whipped into a hard butter-like consistency.

WEED

Weed is a slang term for marijuana that has become more popular than "grass."

CMDA Statement on
Medical Marijuana

In 2019, the Christian Medical & Dental Associations (CMDA) approved the following statement on medical marijuana. This landmark document should be read extensively by all Christian organizations interested in developing policies and guidelines regarding medical marijuana.

The Christian Medical & Dental Associations (CMDA) has developed this policy on "medical marijuana" with both an inherent belief that the Bible is the Word of God--that it speaks into our time and culture and that God gave us his creation to use to its fullest potential—and with the incorporation of scientific evidence which provides a window into the truths about God's creation.

EXECUTIVE SUMMARY

The term "medical marijuana" refers to the insufficiently regulated use of the whole, unprocessed marijuana plant or its extracts to treat symptoms of illness and other conditions. Note that pharmaceutical-grade medications from components of the marijuana plant have been developed according to U.S. Food and Drug Administration (FDA) standards, but these medications are distinct from what is classified here as "medical marijuana." The science supporting "medical marijuana" has been hotly debated and politicized after emerging on state referendums in recent years.

The Bible which is our final authority for faith and practice, speaks to the creation mandate, promotion of the good, and the role of authority. The Bible does not solve every question of policy, but it does provide insights into the use of medical marijuana.

The two main ingredients in marijuana are tetrahydrocannabinol (THC)—the "psychoactive" ingredient, responsible for the euphoria or "high"—and cannabidiol (CBD). Products may contain primarily THC, primarily CBD, or a mixture of both. THC levels are rising substantially in commercially available marijuana, and product containing concentrations greater than 15 percent are being considered for labeling as "hard drugs" in the Netherlands.[1,2]

State legalization of "medical marijuana" has not been accompanied by the rigorous scientific approval process with regulations for dosing, production, packaging and monitoring that have made FDA-approved medications safe and effective. In such states "medical marijuana" is often approved for conditions[3] where research is inadequate.[4] False advertising may mislead vulnerable patients and the public. "Medical" use may inadvertently result in addiction, increased risk of psychosis, mental or psychosocial impairment, lung damage when smoked, and complications for unborn children when used during pregnancy.[4,5] The presence of "medical marijuana" dispensaries may increase access to recreational marijuana for minors.[6] "Medical marijuana" legalization is associated with increased illicit marijuana use,[7] is linked to increased emergency room visits for marijuana-intoxicated children,[8] and has historically been a stepping stone to legalization of recreational marijuana.[9]

CMDA maintains that a reasonable and prudent physician should only recommend FDA-approved pharmaceutical-grade medications when the indications are clear, dosing is well-established, risk-benefit ratios have been investigated and can be applied to individual patients, delivery systems are safe, and careful monitoring is agreed upon. Physicians cannot assume that "medical marijuana" has the labeled amount of active ingredient and is devoid of contaminants and harmful additives. Rather than legalizing a drug by popular vote and political lobbying, CMDA encourages legalization via FDA approval through formal clinical and scientific studies of any marijuana-based therapeutic that has demonstrated medical efficacy and safety by randomized controlled trials. To augment this process, CMDA suggests rescheduling lower potency marijuana to Schedule II[10] to enable medical research into the potential benefits and harms of the use of pharmaceutical-grade marijuana derivatives within established ethical research guidelines. FDA-approved marijuana medications should be prescribed and regulated like any other FDA-approved medication.

A. BIOLOGICAL

1. **Cannabinoids:** The genus *Cannabis* contains cultivars that are commonly referred to as "marijuana." Although over 100 different cannabinoids as well as other compounds have been found in cannabis species, the two main cannabinoids, or active ingredients, are tetrahydrocannabinol (THC) and cannabidiol (CBD).[4] THC is the "psychoactive" ingredient, responsible for the euphoria or "high" that comes from marijuana due to its partial agonist activity on type-1 cannabinoid receptors (CB_1). CB_1 receptors are found in the brain in high concentrations as well as other non-neural tissues such as the gastrointestinal tract and skeletal muscle. A small number of CB_2 receptors are also in the brain.[4] THC's chemical structure is similar to the endogenous cannabinoids (specifically anandamide) which are neurotransmitters that bind to CB receptors.[5] CBD has low affinity for CB_1 and CB_2 receptors and is not psychoactive; it is an agonist of the serotonin 5-HT1A receptor and appears to have anti-inflammatory, antioxidant, and neuroprotective properties.[4] There are THC-type, CBD-type, and hybrid cannabis plants which have predominantly THC, CBD, or a mixture of both cannabinoids, respectively.[4]

2. **"Medical Marijuana":** Cannabis-derived products (dried flowers, resin, oil, sprays, creams, foods, capsules) may be delivered via smoking, inhaling, vaporizing, eating or drinking food products or beverages, topical applications, and suppositories. These products may contain THC alone, CBD alone, or some combination of both.[4] These products are neither FDA-approved nor regulated for consistency in the amount of active compounds or safe processing; they may contain potentially hazardous contaminants or adulterants such as degradation products, microbes, heavy metals, pesticides, fertilizers, glass beads, lead, tobacco, cholinergic compounds, and solvents.[4]

3. **Rising THC Levels:** The natural levels of THC and CBD in Cannabis are under 1%.[11] Using powerful lights, selective breeding, hydration, chemical fertilizers and special soils, the industry has created a new and more potent marijuana plant than the one of the 1960s and 1970s. The average THC content in the "new" marijuana exceeded 12% nationwide in 2014.[5,11] Marijuana concentrates may contain 75% or more THC;[5] associations of the use of such substances with addictive highs, psychosis, and other effects led one author who works in drug treatment programs to claim they are deserving of the label "hard drug,"[11] like heroin and LSD. Although not yet implemented, recommendations have been made to revise the Netherlands Opium Act to place cannabis containing more than 15% THC in List 1 (hard drugs).[1]

B. BIBLICAL

1. **The Bible as our final authority for faith and practice:** We believe the Bi-

ble speaks directly into every social, cultural, and political issue. The Bible does not solve every question of policy, but we do feel it provides insights into the use of medical marijuana.

2. **The Creation mandate:** Genesis relates that God gave humans dominion over all the earth with instructions to subdue it.[12] We have a mandate to use everything our Creator has given us to its fullest potential and greatest good—to God's glory. But the fall[13] caused mankind to begin using creation for selfish and sinful purposes. The marijuana plant has potential good medicinal use for humanity. However, it also has the potential to harm individuals, society, and the environment.

3. **Promotion of the good:** We believe Scripture clearly communicates God's will that people everywhere—in all circumstances—be treated with love, humility, kindness, compassion, and self-control. This means doing good and promoting the good to our neighbors – not evil.[14] CMDA believes society should not approve the use of any medication unless there is (1) a strong evidence-base regarding the efficacy of such drugs in relieving specific symptoms or treating specific medical conditions as validated by a formal regulatory approval pathway, and (2) safe, pharmaceutical-grade, uniform-dosing options available.

4. **Role of authority:** We believe Scripture calls Christians to be submissive to governments and authorities.[15] Since no government or authority is perfect or flawless, there clearly are limits to this submissiveness when the authorities and Biblical commands are in conflict.[16] Leaders and teachers must give an account and are judged more strictly;[17] physicians fill both roles and must be careful never to abuse that authority. Even in states where marijuana is legal for medicinal purposes, the respected authority of the physician's role in society dictates that only FDA-approved, pharmaceutical-grade marijuana be dispensed or prescribed for treatment of conditions for which solid medical evidence of effectiveness exists and for which the benefits exceed potential harms.[18] Cannabis-infused food and plant forms of marijuana have unknown and uncontrollable doses of active components (THC and CBD) and may be unsafely packaged, and therefore should be avoided.

C. SOCIAL

1. **General:** We believe all citizens of a country should consider the known and potential harmful and beneficial effects of marijuana on individuals and society. Experiences with the harms associated with prescription opioids, alcohol, and tobacco are relevant to the consideration of legalizing, prescribing, and dispensing marijuana.

2. **Slippery slope to recreational marijuana use:** The approval of medical marijuana has historically been a stepping stone to approving recreational

marijuana. All states with legal recreational marijuana had prior legalization of medical marijuana.[9] Evidence suggests that overall availability may lead to an increase in recreational usage, which could create a demand for legalization of recreational marijuana. For example, one nationwide study found that medical marijuana laws are associated with "increased prevalence of illicit cannabis use and cannabis use disorders."[7] States with legal medical marijuana have youth rates that surpass those in states that do not.[19] One study from Oregon suggest that communities with a greater number of medical marijuana patients and licensed growers was associated with a higher prevalence of marijuana use among youth from 2006 to 2015. The authors suggest that changing community attitudes in these areas could be influential in teen behavior as well.[6] Other studies have noted equivocal or contrasting findings.[20]such as increased frequency, could be hidden behind the choice of past-month use as a measure; the large surveys on which Sarvet et al's data was extracted may not be representative at the state level; and the changes in attitudes and usage of marijuana in control non-MML states may actually be driven, and thus contaminated by, changes in MML states. (Chu YL. Commentary on Sarvet et al. (2018[21]

3. **Commercialization and social media:** Individuals, small businesses, and corporations who profit from medical marijuana sales are looking to increase its usage. To this end, a variety of advertising venues, including social media platforms, are being used; advertising distortions regarding the benefits of marijuana are not uncommon. For example, in one cross-sectional study in Colorado, almost 70% of contacted marijuana dispensaries recommended cannabis products to treat nausea during pregnancy.[22] Another study examined the website marketing practices of medical and recreational marijuana dispensaries across the U.S., finding that only a few advised about side effects and contraindications. 75% did not include age verification, making products available to youth with convenient online ordering.[23] Exposure to medical marijuana advertising has been associated with greater marijuana use in minors.[24] Physicians should warn their patients about false advertising and youth access.

4. **Opioid addiction:** There has been much hype about marijuana legalization providing a safer replacement for opioid use, with the potential to reduce opioid addiction and overdoses. Evidence is conflicting as to whether this is, in fact, the case,[25] and caution must be used in looking at studies in this area because of bias,[26] unreliability of self-reported use of drugs, the uncertainty of inferring individual substitution behaviors from state-level data relating marijuana legislation and opioid death rates,[27] and other methodological problems. Because societal attitudes may have changed prior to either medical or recreational legalization[6] and because opioid addiction is a complex issue with multiple antecedents that might represent events coinciding with

marijuana legalization, it is difficult to define the associations of legalization of marijuana and opioid use. Samples of research:

a. There are reports that opioid use has increased, rather than decreased, in states legalizing marijuana. In Colorado, for example, opioid use more than doubled among 10 to 19 year-olds after recreational legalization of marijuana.[19]

b. Legalization of marijuana in Colorado is associated with short-term reductions in opioid-related deaths.[28]

c. Medical legalization appears to be associated with "reductions in both prescriptions and dosages of Schedule III (but not Schedule II) opioids received by Medicaid enrollees."[29]

d. A study that examined opioid use in patients following musculoskeletal trauma found that self-reported marijuana use during recovery was associated with an increased amount and duration of opioid use. However, many patients in this study had misperceptions that their marijuana use reduced both their pain and the amount of opioids used.[30]

e. Not only marijuana use but also use of alcohol, illegal methadone, and other opioids was found to increase in pregnant women after legalization of recreational marijuana in Washington State.[31] Cannabis use was associated with an increased risk of developing nonmedical prescription opioid use and opioid use disorder.[32]

D. MEDICAL

1. **Federal Drug Administration (FDA)-Approved Marijuana-Derived Medications:** (pharmaceutical-produced, quality-controlled and dose-specific medications):

    a. **Synthetic THC drugs:** Dronabinol (Marinol and Syndros)[33] and nabilone (Cesamet)[34] have FDA approval for the treatment of chemotherapy-induced nausea and vomiting, and dronabinol is also used to treat loss of appetite and weight in patients with AIDS. A systematic review of anti-nausea efficacy of these medications revealed that side effects were greater and efficacy no better than with the use of traditional anti-nausea medications.[35] These drugs are Schedule II or III (see the Table at the end for a description of scheduling categories).

    b. **Cannabidiol (CBD) drugs:** In June of 2018, the FDA approved the first natural marijuana plant-derived drug, Epidiolex, an oil for the treatment of seizures associated with two rare forms of childhood epilepsy (Lennox-Gastaut and Dravet syndromes).[36] Epidiolex does not contain any THC and has been approved as a Schedule V medication. Schedule V substances are the least restrictive schedule of the Controlled Substances Act.[37] (See the Table at the end for a description of scheduling categories.)

    c.   Currently there are no other FDA-approved uses for any component of the marijuana plant. "Off-label" use of FDA-approved drugs may be indicated in those occasions when the physician determines that there is significant scientific research evidence of benefit that outweighs any potential harm and the patient has failed other FDA-approved therapies; alternatively, there may be appropriate occasions when an FDA-approved drug is used "off-label" in a different form (e.g. oral solution instead of a capsule), for a different (but similar) patient population, or at a different dose.[38]

2. **Studies:** There are a number of concerns with the research in this area:

    a.   **Poor reliability:** The research itself may be unreliable because of factors such as heterogeneity in the active ingredients and contaminants, lack of standard dosing, inadequate research into effects of highly potent types, and variability in the route of consuming marijuana. As an example of the latter, alterations in the number of puffs or volume inhaled may change with the potency of THC in the marijuana being smoked.[39] It is important to note the nature of marijuana derivatives used in any studies—the THC and/or CBD level, delivery method, and quantity. For example, self-reported amount of smoking provides poor data compared to use of FDA-approved standard-dose pharmaceuticals. Conclusive studies can only be done with FDA-regulated medications or pharmaceutical-grade compounds.

    b.   **Regulatory barriers:** Research on marijuana is hampered because of its classification as a Schedule I drug with intimidating bureaucratic regulations to overcome in order to obtain it for research. Much of the federal funding has been earmarked for studying the negative effects of marijuana, and inadequate money is available for investigating potential benefits.[4] Additionally, some academic institutions may fear that conducting research with Schedule I substances could put their federal funding at risk. (See the Table at the end for a description of scheduling categories.)

    c.   **Insufficient data:** In a system proven effective over many decades, medicine aims to establish the safety and effectiveness of treatment by requiring rigorous clinical trials before the FDA will recommend or release medications to large numbers of people. There is a lack of studies on the safety, efficacy, and short-term and long-term effects of marijuana, especially the high potency forms. There are also insufficient studies on the potential drug interactions between cannabis compounds and prescription and non-prescription medications. Researchers, scientific organizations, and representatives of the federal government claim that there is not enough evidence to support the use of marijuana as a beneficial drug and call for more research.[40,41]

  d. **Impediments:** Researcher bias and obtaining properly controlled, adequately-sized, representative samples are among the methodological problems that may be anticipated in this research area.

  e. **Ethical issues:** Adverse health effects of marijuana, especially use of high potency variants and smoking as the means of consumption, highlight ethical problems in exposing research subjects to harm when trying to document the safety or harm of specific consumer products.

  f. **Caution:** Weak or absent evidence about harmful effects of marijuana does not mean they do not exist; caution should be used when even limited evidence suggests a possibility of harm.

3. **Health effects of cannabis use:** A review of the current literature regarding health effects of cannabis, while representing only a snapshot into a rapidly changing landscape and having some limitations, can be found in a recent report from The National Academies of Sciences, Engineering, and Medicine.[4] According to this report, the therapeutic effects of cannabis or cannabinoids are as follows:

  a. **Substantial evidence** of effectiveness for treatment of:

   1) Chronic pain in adults (cannabis)

   2) Antiemetics in chemotherapy-induced nausea and vomiting (oral cannabinoids)

   3) Patient-reported multiple sclerosis spasticity symptoms (oral cannabinoids)

  b. **Moderate evidence** of effectiveness for improving short-term sleep outcomes in patients with sleep disturbances associated with obstructive sleep apnea, fibromyalgia, chronic pain, and multiple sclerosis (cannabinoids, primarily nabiximols[42])

c. **Limited evidence** of effectiveness for:

1) Improving the wasting syndrome associated with HIV/AIDS (cannabis and oral cannabinoids)

2) Clinician-measured multiple sclerosis spasticity symptoms (oral cannabinoids)

3) Symptoms of Tourette syndrome (THC capsules)

4) Improving anxiety symptoms in social anxiety disorders, as assessed by a public speaking test (cannabidiol)

5) Improving symptoms of posttraumatic stress disorder (nabilone—single, small, fair-quality trial)

d. **Limited evidence** of a statistical association between cannabinoids and better outcomes after traumatic brain injury or intracranial hemorrhage

e. **Limited evidence** they are ineffective for:

1) Improving dementia (cannabinoids)

2) Improving intraocular pressure in glaucoma (cannabinoids)

3) Reducing depressive symptoms in patients with chronic pain or multiple sclerosis (nabiximols, dronabinol, and nabilone)

f. **Insufficient evidence** to support or refute the effectiveness of treatment for cancers, cancer-associated anorexia cachexia syndrome and anorexia nervosa, irritable bowel syndrome symptoms, epilepsy, spasticity due to spinal cord injury paralysis, symptoms of amyotrophic lateral sclerosis, chorea and certain symptoms of Huntington's disease, motor symptoms of Parkinson's disease, levodopa-induced dyskinesis, and dystonia.

4. **Medical complications of marijuana use:** Despite the lack of research, some of the short-term and long-term effects of marijuana use are being uncovered. In all associations or lack thereof of marijuana use and health complications listed below, the conclusions are often drawn in the face of insufficient good quality and conflicting data and with the knowledge that research may not reflect the current products being used by consumers. Therefore, future research will be needed to provide more definitive answers to questions about effects of marijuana use.

a. **Cancer:** There is limited evidence of a statistical association between current, frequent, or chronic cannabis smoking and one type of testicular tumor, but not current sufficient evidence of associations between marijuana use and other cancer types in adults. There is minimal evidence that cannabis use during pregnancy is associated with a greater risk of cancer in offspring.[4]

b. **Respiratory diseases:** There is substantial evidence of an association between chronic marijuana smoking and chronic bronchitis and worsening respiratory symptoms.[43] There is more limited evidence of an association with chronic obstructive pulmonary disease (COPD).[4]

c. **Injury and death:** Substantial evidence correlates cannabis use and increased risk of motor vehicle crashes.[4]

d. **Pre-and perinatal exposure to maternal cannabis use:** Use of marijuana during pregnancy increased in Washington State after legalization,[31] and is on the rise nationally.[44] According to a recent study, nearly 70 percent of approved marijuana dispensaries in Colorado recommended marijuana to pregnant mothers experiencing morning sickness.[22] Marijuana has potentially serious effects on the developing fetus.[44-46] A recent study documented that prenatal THC exposure adversely affects infant neurobehavior and child development up through the teen years,[47] but other researchers feel data is lacking to draw conclusions about long-term effects.[4] Overall review of current studies suggests a substantial association between maternal smoking of marijuana with lower birth weight babies and more limited evidence of a correlation with pregnancy complications for the mother and admission of the newborn to intensive care.[4]

e. **Teen use:** Heavy marijuana use can damage brain development in youth ages 13 to 18. There is evidence of an association between cannabis use and loss of concentration and memory, jumbled thinking, schizophrenia, and early onset paranoid psychosis.[48]

f. **Psychosocial impairment:** Moderate evidence correlates acute cannabis use with impaired learning, memory, and attention, and more limited evidence suggests that such impairments may be neurotoxic in that effects are sustained even after prolonged abstinence from cannabis use.[4,49,50] More limited associations exist between cannabis use and impaired academic achievement and outcomes, higher unemployment, lower income, and impaired social functioning.[4] Neurocognitive effects also include a decline in IQ, memory problems, and attentional impairments.[49,50]

g. **Mental health:** There is substantial evidence of statistical association between cannabis use and the development of schizophrenia and other psychoses,[51] with greater risk occurring among more frequent users.[4] In two studies of patients with drug-induced psychosis (most or all being cannabis as the inciting drug), one-third to one-half of the patients later developed a schizophrenia-spectrum disorder.[52,53] Those with drug-induced psychosis were equally as violent as schizophrenia patients who misused drugs.[52] Moderate evidence associates cannabis use with increased incidence of developing depression; suicidal ideation, attempts, and completion; and social anxiety disorder. More limited evidence links cannabis use with certain increased symptoms (e.g. hallucinations) in psychotic disorders, development of bipolar disorder, the development and/or increased symptoms of anxiety disorders, and increased symptoms of posttraumatic stress disorder.[4]

h. **High doses or use of some high potency and/or synthetic cannabis derivatives** have produced the following effects: psychosis, mood alterations, panic attacks, cognitive impairment, dizziness, cardiovascular effects (tachycardia, hypertension, palpitations), nausea, appetite changes, and others.[5] Mental impairment and distressing emotional states, such as paranoia, hallucinations, and psychosis, have caused people to harm themselves and others.[52,54,55]

i. **Addiction:** Use of marijuana can become problematic (marijuana use disorder) which may progress to addiction in some cases; when a person cannot stop using the drug despite interference with many aspects of daily life, use disorder is classified as addiction.[5] A 2015 study suggests that "30 percent of those who use marijuana may have some degree of marijuana use disorder."[5] Marijuana use disorder is frequently "associated with dependence—in which a person feels withdrawal symptoms when not taking the drug."[5] A user may be dependent but not be addicted. Studies estimate that 9 percent of adults[56] and 17 percent of teens who use marijuana will become dependent on it.[5] In 2015 roughly 4 million people in the US were found to have a marijuana use disorder, and 138,000 sought treatment.[5] In the same year in the Netherlands, more first-time entrants and more people overall entered treatment programs for cannabis use than for any other drug.[1] Although modulation of smoking technique may partially blunt the effect of use of high potency cannabis,[39] there is evidence that higher potency marijuana use is associated with increased severity of cannabis dependence.[57] There is moderate evidence of an association between cannabis use and the development of substance dependence and/ or a substance abuse disorder for other substances, including tobacco, alcohol, and illegal drugs.[4,58]

j. **Delivery method:** Smoking is a harmful route of administration for any medicinal compound because of carcinogens and other harmful materials which are known to produce adverse effects on the lungs and other tissues. Marijuana joints may contain "particulate matter, toxic gases, reactive oxygen species, and polycyclic aromatic hydrocarbons at a concentration possibly 20 times that of tobacco smoke."[59] Histopathologic changes in bronchial inflammation that are similar to changes seen with smoking tobacco have been found in marijuana smokers.[59] Only other delivery methods of FDA-approved cannabis compounds should be prescribed.

5. **Inaccurate public analysis and use of research:** Current state medical marijuana laws specifically approve medical marijuana as treatment for illnesses such as HIV, ALS, hepatitis, Parkinson's cancer, and glaucoma,[3] even though the data from scientific studies is weak or even nonexistent in most of these diseases.[4] As an example, multiple states include ALS on their list of approved illnesses for medical marijuana, but there have been only two small randomized double-blind clinical studies and the results of effectiveness were unequivocally negative.[4] Washington D.C. does not restrict medical marijuana use to any specific disease.[3,60] While scientific studies may eventually show benefit from cannabinoids for some of these illnesses, that is clearly not the case at this time. As a result, vulnerable and suffering patients are being misled and deceived.

6. **Physician response to "medical marijuana":**

   a. **Irresponsible behavior:** One study found almost one half of cancer doctors say they have recently recommended medical marijuana to their patients, although 70 percent of them admitted they did not have sufficient knowledge to do so.[61] Marijuana should not be discussed with, or prescribed to, patients without clear evidence-based guidelines supporting its use.

   b. **Responsible behavior:** The Cleveland Clinic and other reputable hospitals have prohibited physicians on staff from recommending "medical marijuana."[62] Dr. Paul Terpeluk, Medical Director at the Cleveland Clinic, summarizes why it does not make sense for physicians to prescribe it: "In the world of healthcare, a medication is a drug that has endured extensive clinical trials, public hearings and approval by the U.S. Food & Drug Administration (FDA). Medications are tested for safety and efficacy. They are closely regulated, from production to distribution. They are accurately dosed, down to the milligram. Medical marijuana is none of those things."[63]

E. LEGAL AND PRACTICAL IMPLICATIONS

1. **Marijuana classification:** The U.S. still classifies marijuana in the same category as heroin, as a Schedule I Drug, which has "no currently accepted medical use and a high potential for abuse."[64] The United States Food and Drug Administration (FDA) does not recognize, regulate, or approve the marijuana plant as medicine. They state: "researchers haven't conducted enough large-scale clinical trials that show that the benefits of the marijuana plant (as opposed to its cannabinoid ingredients) outweigh its risks in patients it's meant to treat."[25] Because of the vast increase in marijuana potency and the potential for harm and addiction, there is a need for limiting access to marijuana. When medical benefits are established for FDA-approved, pharmaceutical-grade derivatives of marijuana, these substances have been classified as Schedule II (Syndros), III (Marinol),[65] or V (Epidiolex).[37] (See the Table at the end for a description of scheduling categories.)

2. **State regulations:** As of late 2018, thirty-three states, the District of Columbia, Guam and Puerto Rico have approved medical marijuana.[9] Klieger et al evaluated laws in 28 states (including the District of Columbia) that had approved "medical marijuana," as of February 2017.[60] Besides specifying different qualifying diseases, the states varied in protections for patients against discrimination, in requirements for product safety testing, and in the range of packaging and labeling regulations.[60] Enforcement and adequacy of state regulations is unclear. Although Colorado, for example, has packaging regulations,[60] the number of children under 12 with marijuana ingestion visits to emergency rooms went from 0% to 2.4% of total visits after medical marijuana legalization.[8] After recreational marijuana was legalized in 2014 in Colorado, increases in pediatric hospital visits and calls to poison control due to marijuana ingestion have continued to increase,[66,67] with hospital visits doubling in 2017.[67] The majority of exposures were due to ingestion of medical marijuana in a food product.[8,66,67] State referenda approving the use of "medical marijuana," essentially a form of potentially addictive and harmful herbal therapy, with the inability to monitor or control the dose of active compounds, without clear safety standards or clinical guidelines,[60] and in the absence of evidence of effectiveness and a positive risk/benefit ratio, is unique in modern medicine.

3. **Legal dichotomy:** When medical marijuana is legally allowed in a state, the state has agreed to allow consumers to purchase marijuana from regulated dispensaries if they have a physician's prescription. However, because marijuana is a Schedule I Drug, physicians who prescribe medical marijuana (non-pharmaceutical grade, non-standard dose, non-FDA-approved mar-

ijuana) from dispensaries are violating federal law, even if they are in compliance with state law. FDA-approved pharmaceutical grade standard dose medications derived from marijuana (e.g. Marinol) are legal in all states and physicians may prescribe them for appropriate indications and patients. The FDA cannot regulate marijuana edibles or any other forms of "medical marijuana" because marijuana is illegal; standard dosing and safety of these potentially pesticide and chemical-laden products[4] are illusory.

4. **Practical recommendations:** Rescheduling lower potency marijuana to Schedule II to make research easier and to allow FDA involvement in regulating marijuana on a national, rather than state, level seems reasonable. (See the Table at the end for a description of scheduling categories.) There should not be a double standard for prescription medications. All need to be subject to FDA regulations for safety of consumers and the respectability of the medical profession.

F. CMDA RECOMMENDATIONS FOR CHRISTIAN HEALTHCARE PROFESSIONALS

1. CMDA maintains that a reasonable and prudent physician should only recommend FDA-approved medications when the indications are clear, dosing is well-established, risk benefit ratios have been investigated and can be applied to individual patients, delivery systems are safe, and careful monitoring is agreed upon.

2. State legalization of "medical marijuana" has not been accompanied by the rigorous scientific approval process with regulations for dosing, production, packaging and monitoring that have made FDA-approved medications safe and effective. State-approved dispensaries are marketing a form of potentially addictive and harmful herbal therapy that does not meet modern safety and efficacy standards or clinical guidelines. Physicians cannot assume that "medical marijuana" is safe or effective for state-listed qualifying diseases or conditions, nor can they be sure that it has the labeled amount of active ingredient and is devoid of contaminants and harmful additives.

3. There are risks of significant short-term and long-term complications associated with marijuana use, including addiction; medical, mental health, psychosocial, and cognitive problems; and increasing the likelihood of problems for the unborn, children, and teens. These risks should make any medical use of marijuana a serious decision in which benefits clearly outweigh the risks. Given the inadequate research on marijuana benefits and the few conditions for which there are even moderate or better evidence of effectiveness (often accompanied by significant side effects), indications for prescribing marijuana are limited at this time.

4. Rather than legalizing marijuana for medical use by popular vote and political lobbying, CMDA encourages legalization via FDA approval through formal clinical and scientific studies of any marijuana-based therapeutic that has demonstrated medical efficacy and safety by randomized controlled trials. To augment this process, CMDA supports rescheduling lower potency marijuana to Schedule II to enable medical research into the potential benefits and harms of the use of pharmaceutical-grade marijuana derivatives within established ethical research guidelines and FDA supervision.

5. CMDA recommends that FDA-approved marijuana medications should be regulated and regarded like any other FDA-approved medication. Medications that have been approved by the FDA have been studied extensively and have undergone a lengthy and rigorous process before they are made available to the public. The FDA requires carefully conducted studies (clinical trials) in hundreds to thousands of human subjects to determine the benefits and risks of a possible medication. These medications have carefully regulated manufacturing processes, quality and purity standards, and standardized dosing and prescribing requirements.

G. CMDA RECOMMENDATIONS FOR THE CHRISTIAN COMMUNITY

Because of inadequate research, potential addiction and health hazards of marijuana use, inadequate regulation in state laws to ensure safety and efficacy, and misleading advertising, CMDA recommends the following:

1. Most medical conditions are best treated with FDA-approved medications that are devoid of addictive qualities and significant complications. Indications for prescribing marijuana are limited, and medications with fewer risks are the first line of therapy. However, in cases where primary treatments have not been adequate, and a trial of THC or CBD compounds might be considered, seek medical care from a qualified health professional who can prescribe currently available, pharmaceutical-grade, FDA-approved marijuana derivatives for appropriate conditions with proper monitoring.

2. Be wary of claims made about marijuana "benefits."

3. "Medical marijuana" dispensaries may have products with unknown contaminants and additives, variable amounts of active ingredients, unproven efficacy, unclear short-term and long-term problems, and unsafe packaging. This is not medicine.

4. Smoking any product is never healthy and should not be considered "medicine."

5. Be vigilant to ensure that children do not inadvertently have access to "medical marijuana" when visiting or in someone else's care.

6. Encourage federal government authorities to change lower potency marijuana to Schedule II to enable better research to elucidate potential benefits and harms of pharmaceutical grade marijuana products under the auspices of the FDA.

Approved by the Board of Trustees – February 20, 2019

Controlled Substances Act Scheduling	
Schedule	Description of substances
I	No accepted medical use and a high potential for abuse
II	High potential for abuse with risk of severe psychological or physical dependence
III	Moderate to low potential for physical and psychological dependence. Abuse potential less than Schedule I and II, but more than IV.
IV	Low potentials for abuse and risk of dependence.
V	Lower potential for abuse than Schedule IV; preparations containing limited quantities of certain narcotics. Generally used for antidiarrheal, antitussive, and analgesic purposes.
Examples	
Heroin, LSD, marijuana	
Vicodin, hydromorphone, meperidine, cocaine, fentanyl, Ritalin	
Products with < 90mg codeine per dose (Tylenol with codeine), ketamine, anabolic steroids	
Xanax, Soma, Darvon, Valium, Ativan, Ambien, Tramadol	
Cough preparations with < 200 mg codeine or per 100 mL (Robitussin AC), Lomotil, Motofen, Lyrica, Parepectolin	

Adapted from: DEA. Drug Scheduling. *https://www.dea.gov/drug-scheduling* (accessed Feb. 7, 2019)

REFERENCES AND BIBLIOGRAPHY

1   European Monitoring Centre for Drugs and Drug Addiction. Netherlands Country Drug Report 2017. Luxembourg: Publications Office of the European Union; 2017.

2   Lemmens P. Dutch government pressured to reconsider planned re-scheduling of cannabis in drug law. *Addiction* 2014; 109(10): 1761-2.

3   Compassionate Certification Centers. List of Qualifying Health Conditions For Medical Marijuana In Each State. October 26, 2017. *https://www.compassionatecertification-centers.com/list-of-qualifying-health-conditions-for-medical-marijuana-in-each-state/* (accessed Feb. 5 2019).

4   National Academies of Sciences Engineering and Medicine. The Health Effects of Cannabis and Cannabinoids: The Current State of Evidence and Recommendations for Research. Washington, DC: The National Academies Press; 2017.

5   National Institute on Drug Abuse. Marijuana. June 2018. *https://d14rmgtrwzf5a. cloudfront.net/sites/default/files/1380-marijuana.pdf.*

6   Paschall MJ, Grube JW, Biglan A. Medical marijuana legalization and marijuana use among youth in Oregon. *The Journal of Primary Prevention* 2017; 38(3): 329-41.

7   Hasin DS, Sarvet AL, Cerda M, et al. US Adult Illicit Cannabis Use, Cannabis Use Disorder, and Medical Marijuana Laws 1991-1992 to 2012-2013. *JAMA Psychiatry* 2017; 74(6): 579-88.

8   Wang GS, Roosevelt G, Heard K. Pediatric Marijuana Exposures in a Medical Marijuana State. *JAMA Pediatrics* 2013; 167(7): 630-3.

9   National Conference of State Legislatures. State Medical Marijuana Laws. 1/23/2019. *http://www.ncsl.org/research/health/state-medical-marijuana-laws.aspx* (accessed Feb. 3 2019).

10 See the Table at the end of the statement for a description of drug scheduling categories.

11 Cort B. Weed, Inc. : the truth about THC, the pot lobby, and the commercial marijuana industry. Deerfield Beach, Florida: Health Communications, Inc.; 2017.

12 Genesis 1:28

13 Genesis 3

14 Matthew 22:36-40

15 Romans 13

16 Daniel 3

17 Hebrews 13:17 and James 3:1

18 Hiippocratic Oath and Matthew 22: 36-40

19 Smart Approaches to Marijuana. Lessons Learned From Marijuana Legalization, 2018. *https://learnaboutsam.org/wp-content/uploads/2018/07/SAM-Lessons-Learned-From-Marijuana-Legalization-Digital-1.pdf.*

20 A meta-analysis of 11 studies from four large national surveys compared adolescents' past-month marijuana use prevalence pre-and post- changes in state medical marijuana laws (MMLs). Comparison between pre-post MML changes in MML states to changes in non-MML states over comparable time periods yielded non-significant differences between changes in adolescents' past month use prevalence in the two states.(Sarvet AL, Wall MM, Fink DS, et al. Medical marijuana laws and adolescent marijuana use in the United States: a systematic review and meta-analysis. *Addiction* 2018; 113(6): 1003-16.) However, Chu argues that caution is indicated in accepting

this conclusion for the following reasons: changes in other measurements of marijuana use, such as increased frequency, could be hidden behind the choice of past-month use as a measure; the large surveys on which Sarvet et al's data was extracted may not be representative at the state level; and the changes in attitudes and usage of marijuana in control non-MML states may actually be driven, and thus contaminated by, changes in MML states.(Chu YL. Commentary on Sarvet et al. (2018): What do we still need to know about the impacts of medical marijuana laws in the United States? *Addiction* 2018; 113(6): 1017-8.)

21 A study comparing pre-post MML differences in teen use of marijuana, cigarettes, binge drinking, and other illicit or non-prescribed drugs found that MML enactment was associated with a decrease in the use of such substances for early adolescents, no change for 10th graders, but an increase in non-medical prescription opioid and cigarette use among 12th graders. The authors suggested that parents of younger children may have been more vigilant about warning about marijuana use after MML passage; limitations to their study were also discussed. Limitations include: substance use was self-reported, study only included school-attending adolescents, specific features of MMLs were not assessed, assumption that the passage of MML in one state did not affect the behaviors of individuals in nearby, non-MML states (perhaps this assumption is incorrect), concurrent policy changes may have confounded the relationships of interest.(Cerdá M, Sarvet AL, Wall M, et al. Medical marijuana laws and adolescent use of marijuana and other substances: Alcohol, cigarettes, prescription drugs, and other illicit drugs. *Drug & Alcohol Dependence* 2018; 183: 62-8.)

22 Dickson B, Mansfield C, Guiahi M, et al. Recommendations From Cannabis Dispensaries About First-Trimester Cannabis Use. *Obstetrics & Gynecology* 2018; 131(6): 1031-8.

23 Cavazos-Rehg PA, Krauss MJ, Cahn E, et al. Marijuana Promotion Online: an Investigation of Dispensary Practices. *Prev Sci* 2018.

24 D'Amico EJ, Rodriguez A, Tucker JS, Pedersen ER, Shih RA, D'Amico EJ. Planting the seed for marijuana use: Changes in exposure to medical marijuana advertising and subsequent adolescent marijuana use, cognitions, and consequences over seven years. *Drug & Alcohol Dependence* 2018; 188: 385-91.

25 National Institute on Drug Abuse. What is medical marijuana? June 2018 June 2018. *https://www.drugabuse.gov/publications/drugfacts/marijuana-medicine* (accessed February 5 2019).

26 Example of bias: An article by Lucas (Lucas P. Rationale for cannabis-based interventions in the opioid overdose crisis. *Harm Reduction Journal* 2017; 14: 1-6) advocated for medical and recreational legalization of marijuana as a way to reduce opioid addiction and overdoses. However, the Methods section did not reveal the mechanism of article selection nor any other methods, no conflicting data was mentioned at all, and the author's conflict of interest was noted in small print at the end of the article—he is VP and stockholder with a federally authorized medical cannabis production & research company in Canada.

27 Caputi TL, Sabet KA. Population-level analyses cannot tell us anything about individual-level marijuana-opioid substitution. *American Journal of Public Health* 2018; 108(3): e12-e.

28 Livingston MD, Barnett TE, Delcher C, Wagenaar AC. Recreational Cannabis Le-

galization and Opioid-Related Deaths in Colorado, 2000-2015. *American Journal of Public Health* 2017; 107(11): 1827-9.

29 Liang D, Bao Y, Wallace M, Grant I, Shi Y. Medical cannabis legalization and opioid prescriptions: evidence on US Medicaid enrollees during 1993-2014. *Addiction* 2018; 113(11): 2060-70.

30 Bhashyam AR, Heng M, Harris MB, Vrahas MS, Weaver MJ. Self-Reported Marijuana Use Is Associated with Increased Use of Prescription Opioids Following Traumatic Musculoskeletal Injury. *J Bone Joint Surg Am* 2018; 100(24): 2095-102.

31 Grant TM, Graham JC, Carlini BH, Ernst CC, Brown NN. Use of marijuana and other substances among pregnant and parenting women with substance use disorders: Changes in Washington state after marijuana legalization. *Journal of Studies on Alcohol and Drugs* 2018; 79(1): 88-95.

32 Olfson M, Wall MM, Shang-Min L, Blanco C. Cannabis Use and Risk of Prescription Opioid Use Disorder in the United States. *American Journal of Psychiatry* 2018; 175(1): 47-53.

33 *https://medlineplus.gov/druginfo/meds/a607054.html*. Accessed Jan. 10, 2019.

34 *https://medlineplus.gov/druginfo/meds/a607048.html*. Accessed Feb. 4, 2019

35 Smith LA, Azariah F, Lavender VTC, Stoner NS, Bettiol S. Cannabinoids for nausea and vomiting in adults with cancer receiving chemotherapy. *Cochrane Database of Systematic Reviews* 2015; (11).

36 *https://medlineplus.gov/druginfo/meds/a618051.html*. Accessed Jan. 10, 2019.

37 United States Drug Enforcement Administration. FDA-approved drug Epidiolex placed in schedule V of Controlled Substance Act. September 27, 2018. *https://www.dea.gov/press-releases/2018/09/27/fda-approved-drug-epidiolex-placed-schedule-v-controlled-substance-act* (accessed Feb. 4 2019).

38 U.S. Food and Drug Administration. Understanding Unapproved Use of Approved Drugs "Off Label". 2/05/2018. *https://www.fda.gov/forpatients/other/offlabel/default.htm* (accessed Feb. 4 2019).

39 Pol P, Liebregts N, Brunt T, et al. Cross-sectional and prospective relation of cannabis potency, dosing and smoking behaviour with cannabis dependence: an ecological study. *Addiction* 2014; 109(7): 1101-9.

40 The National Academies of Sciences, Engineering and Medicine recently called on the federal government to support better research, decrying the "lack of definitive evidence on using medical marijuana." U.S. Secretary of Health and Human Services Alex Azar recently said there was "no such thing as medical marijuana." (Wedell K. "No such thing as medical marijuana," Health Secretary says. Dayton Daily News. 2018 March 2.)

41 Carney JK. Brief Commentary: Advocating for Blunt Policy. *Annals of Internal Medicine* 2019; 170(2): 121-.

42 An oromucosal spray containing both THC and CBD. It also has a brand name of Sativex and is on the FDA Fast Track for approval. (National Academies of Sciences Engineering and Medicine. The Health Effects of Cannabis and Cannabinoids: The Current State of Evidence and Recommendations for Research. Washington, DC: The National Academies Press; 2017.)

43 Tashkin DP. Marijuana and Lung Disease. *CHEST* 2018; 154(3): 653-63.

44 Adashi EY. Brief Commentary: Marijuana Use During Gestation and Lactation—

Harmful Until Proved Safe Marijuana Use During Gestation and Lactation. *Annals of Internal Medicine* 2019; 170(2): 122-.

45 Volkow ND, Compton WM, Wargo EM. The Risks of Marijuana Use During Pregnancy. *JAMA* 2017; 317(2): 129-30.

46 Grant KS, Petroff R, Isoherranen N, Stella N, Burbacher TM. Cannabis use during pregnancy: Pharmacokinetics and effects on child development. *Pharmacol Ther* 2018; 182: 133-51.

47 Jansson LM, Jordan CJ, Velez ML. Perinatal Marijuana Use and the Developing Child. *JAMA: Journal of the American Medical Association* 2018; 320(6): 545-6.

48 Dr. Phil Tibbo, one of the leaders in the medical field and initiator of Nova Scotia's Weed Myths campaign targeting teens, has seen firsthand evidence of what heavy use can do as director of Nova Scotia's Early Psychosis Program. His brain research shows that regular marijuana use leads to an increased risk of developing psychosis and schizophrenia, effectively exploding popular and rather blasé notions that marijuana is "harmless" to teens and "recreational use" is simply "fun and healthy." Multiple researchers have all come to the same conclusion: the younger the brain, the worse the effects in both the short-term and long-term. (Tibbo P, Crocker CE, Lam RW, Meyer J, Sareen J, Aitchison KJ. Implications of Cannabis Legalization on Youth and Young Adults. *Canadian Journal of Psychiatry* 2018; 63(1): 65-71.)

49 Harvey PD. Smoking Cannabis and Acquired Impairments in Cognition: Starting Early Seems Like a Really Bad Idea. *Am J Psychiatry* 2019; 176(2): 90-1.

50 Morin J-FG, Afzali MH, Bourque J, et al. A Population-Based Analysis of the Relationship Between Substance Use and Adolescent Cognitive Development. *American Journal of Psychiatry* 2019; 176(2): 98-106.

51 Malone DT, Hill MN, Rubino T. Adolescent cannabis use and psychosis: epidemiology and neurodevelopmental models. *British Journal of Pharmacology* 2010; 160(3): 511-22.

52 Crebbin K, Mitford E, Paxton R, Turkington D. First-episode drug-induced psychosis: A medium term follow up study reveals a high-risk group. *Social Psychiatry and Psychiatric Epidemiology* 2009; 44(9): 710-5.

53 Arendt M, Rosenberg R, Foldager L, Perto G, Munk-Jørgensen P. Cannabis-induced psychosis and subsequent schizophrenia-spectrum disorders: Follow-up study of 535 incident cases. *The British Journal of Psychiatry* 2005; 187(6): 510-5.

54 Korkmaz Sshc, Turhan L, İzci F, Sağlam S, Atmaca M. Sociodemographic and clinical characteristics of patients with violence attempts with psychotic disorders. *European Journal of General Medicine* 2017; 14(4): 94-8.

55 Douglas KS, Guy LS, Hart SD. Psychosis as a Risk Factor for Violence to Others: A Meta-Analysis. *Psychological Bulletin;* 2009. p. 679-706.

56 Lopez-Quintero C, Perez de los Cobos J, Hasin DS, et al. Probability and predictors of transition from first use to dependence on nicotine, alcohol, cannabis, and cocaine: Results of the National Epidemiologic Survey on Alcohol and Related Conditions (NESARC). *Drug and Alcohol Dependence* 2011; 115(1-2): 120-30.

57 Freeman TP, Winstock AR. Examining the profile of high-potency cannabis and its association with severity of cannabis dependence. *Psychological Medicine* 2015; 45(15): 3181-9.

58 Blanco C, Hasin DS, Wall MM, et al. Cannabis use and risk of psychiatric disorders:

Prospective evidence from a US national longitudinal study. *JAMA Psychiatry* 2016; 73(4): 388-95.

59 Caviedes I, Labarca G, Silva CF, Fernandez-Bussy S. Marijuana Use, Respiratory Symptoms, and Pulmonary Function. *Annals of Internal Medicine* 2019; 170(2): 142-.

60 Klieger SB, Gutman A, Allen L, Pacula RL, Ibrahim JK, Burris S. Mapping medical marijuana: state laws regulating patients, product safety, supply chains and dispensaries, 2017. *Addiction* 2017; 112(12): 2206-16.

61 Braun IM, Wright A, Peteet J, et al. Medical Oncologists' Beliefs, Practices, and Knowledge Regarding Marijuana Used Therapeutically: A Nationally Representative Survey Study. *J Clin Oncol* 2018; 36(19): 1957-62.

62 Hancock L. Cleveland Clinic, UH, MetroHealth staff docs prohibited from recommending medical marijuana. 2018 November 15.

63 Terpeluk P. Should "Medical Marijuana" Be Recommended for Patients? Why our answer is "no". Jan. 10 2019. *https://health.clevelandclinic.org/should-medical-marijuana-be-recommended-for-patients/?utm_campaign=cc+posts&utm_medium=social&utm_source=facebook&utm_content=190107+medical&cvosrc=social+network.facebook.cc+posts&cvo_creative=190107+medical* (accessed Jan. 12 2019).

64 DEA. Drug Scheduling. *https://www.dea.gov/drug-scheduling* (accessed Jan. 4, 2019 2019).

65 *https://www.deadiversion.usdoj.gov/schedules/orangebook/c_cs_alpha.pdf*. Accessed Feb. 5, 2019

66 Wang GS, Le Lait M-C, Deakyne SJ, Bronstein AC, Bajaj L, Roosevelt G. Unintentional Pediatric Exposures to Marijuana in Colorado, 2009-2015. *JAMA Pediatrics* 2016; 170(9): Article.

67 Wang GS, Hoyte C, Roosevelt G, Heard K. The Continued Impact of Marijuana Legalization on Unintentional Pediatric Exposures in Colorado. *Clinical Pediatrics* 2019; 58(1): 114-6.

CMDA Statement on Recreational Marijuana

In 2019, the Christian Medical & Dental Associations (CMDA) approved the following statement on medical marijuana. This landmark document should be read extensively by all Christian organizations interested in developing policies and guidelines regarding medical marijuana.

The Christian Medical & Dental Associations (CMDA) has developed this policy on "recreational marijuana" with both an inherent belief that the Bible is the Word of God—that it speaks into our time and culture and that God gave us His creation to use to its fullest potential—and with the incorporation of scientific evidence which provides a window into the truths about God's creation.

EXECUTIVE SUMMARY

The term "recreational marijuana" refers to any form of marijuana, its derivatives, or synthetic derivatives used for recreational, non-medical purposes. Marijuana has been in the news constantly as American states and countries around the world have been asked to make important decisions about the decriminalization, legalization, and regulation of recreational marijuana.

The Bible is our final authority for faith and practice which speaks to the creation mandate, promotion of the good, the role of authority, and being good stewards of the environment. The Bible does not solve every question of policy, but it does provide insight into the use of recreational marijuana.

The two main cannabinoids, or active ingredients, in marijuana are tetrahydrocannabinol, also called THC, and cannabidiol, or CBD. Cannabis-derived products (dried flowers, resin, oil, sprays, creams, foods, capsules) may be delivered via smoking, inhaling, vaporizing, eating or drinking food products or beverages, topical applications, and suppositories. THC is the euphoria-producing component sought by recreational users and levels have been steadily rising in marijuana plants and products. Recreational marijuana is federally illegal and is neither FDA-approved nor regulated.

Recreational marijuana use and legalization have profound social implications, including associated increases in the following: accidents and death, access to marijuana for minors, crime, drug use and abuse, black market activity, and environmental problems. Low income populations may be affected at a higher incidence than others. The cost to society of recreational marijuana legalization is greater than tax revenues produced from its sales.

Because marijuana has been illegal in the United States until its recent, selective legalization in multiple states, and because it remains illegal federally, high-quality research regarding the safety or risks associated with current recreationally-used marijuana products (especially those containing high levels of THC) is sparse. However, a lack of studies on such products does not mean risk is absent. On the contrary, there is moderate to substantial evidence of health hazards with marijuana use, including associations with respiratory problems (when smoked), motor vehicle crashes, mental or psychosocial problems, increased incidence of schizophrenia and other mental health problems, and addiction. Maternal marijuana smoking is also associated with complications for unborn children. Future research on higher level THC products has the potential to demonstrate even more harm.

For these reasons, CMDA does not support the legalization or use of recreational marijuana. CMDA maintains that healthcare professionals should abstain and strongly advise against the use of recreational marijuana.

A. BIOLOGICAL

1. **Cannabinoids:** The genus *Cannabis* contains cultivars that are commonly referred to as "marijuana." Although over 100 different cannabinoids as well as other compounds have been found in cannabis species, the two main cannabinoids, or active ingredients, are tetrahydrocannabinol (THC) and cannabidiol (CBD).[1] THC is the "psychoactive" ingredient, responsible for the euphoria or "high" that comes from marijuana due to its partial agonist

activity on type-1 cannabinoid receptors (CB1). CB1 receptors are found in the brain in high concentrations as well as other non-neural tissues such as the gastrointestinal tract and skeletal muscle. A small number of CB2 receptors are also in the brain.[1] THC's chemical structure is similar to the endogenous cannabinoids (specifically anandamide) which are neurotransmitters that bind to CB receptors.[2] CBD has low affinity for CB1 and CB2 receptors and is not psychoactive; it is an agonist of the serotonin 5-HT1A receptor and appears to have anti-inflammatory, antioxidant, and neuroprotective properties.[1] There are THC-type, CBD-type, and hybrid cannabis plants which have predominantly THC, CBD, or a mixture of both cannabinoids, respectively.[1]

2. **Marijuana products:** Cannabis-derived products (dried flowers, resin, oil, sprays, creams, foods, capsules) may be delivered via smoking, inhaling, vaporizing, eating or drinking food products or beverages, topical applications, and suppositories. These products may contain THC alone, CBD alone, or some combination of both.[1] Often the products produced for "medical" use are the same as those used recreationally, with the exception that recreational products always contain THC, which produces the "high." These products are neither FDA-approved nor regulated for consistency in the amount of active compounds or safe processing; they may contain potentially hazardous contaminants or adulterants such as degradation products, microbes, heavy metals, pesticides, fertilizers, glass beads, lead, tobacco, cholinergic compounds, and solvents.[1]

3. **Rising THC Levels:** The natural levels of THC and CBD in Cannabis are under 1%.[3] Using powerful lights, selective breeding, hydration, chemical fertilizers and special soils, the industry has created a new and more potent marijuana plant than the one of the 1960s and 1970s. The average THC content in the "new" marijuana exceeded 12% nationwide in 2014.[2,3] Marijuana concentrates may contain 75% or more THC;[2] associations of the use of such substances with addictive highs, psychosis, and other effects led one author who works in drug treatment programs to claim they are deserving of the label "hard drug,"[3] like heroin and LSD. Although not yet implemented, recommendations have been made to revise the Netherlands Opium Act to place cannabis containing more than 15% THC in List 1 (hard drugs).[4]

B. BIBLICAL

1. **The Bible as our final authority for faith and practice:** We believe the Bible speaks directly into every social, cultural, and political issue. The Bible does not solve every question of policy or ethics, but it provides insights into the use of recreational marijuana.

2. **The Creation mandate:** Genesis relates that God gave humans dominion over all the earth with instructions to subdue it.[5] We have a mandate to use everything our Creator has given us to its fullest potential and greatest good—to God's glory. But the fall[6] caused mankind to begin using creation for selfish and sinful purposes. The marijuana plant has potential good medicinal use for humanity. However, it also has the potential to harm individuals, society, and the environment.

3. **Promotion of the Good:** We believe Scripture clearly communicates God's will that people everywhere—in all circumstances—be treated with love, humility, kindness, compassion, and self-control. This means doing good and promoting the good to our neighbors – not evil.[7] Society should not condone harmful behaviors including the promotion and use of hallucinogenic, potentially addicting drugs, like marijuana. Scripture cautions us to not be mastered by anything,[8] for when anything or person other than God is master, we are guilty of idolatry[9] in not loving God with all of our heart, mind, body, and soul.[10]

4. **Biblical admonitions against an altered state of mind:** Multiple passages label drunkenness as sin and an undesirable behavior.[11] Because an altered state of mind is intrinsic to marijuana use, it should not be used for recreational purposes.[12]

5. **Role of authority:** We believe Scripture calls Christians to be submissive to governments and authorities.[13] Since no government or authority is perfect or flawless, there clearly are limits to this submissiveness when the authorities and Biblical commands are in conflict.[14] Leaders and teachers must give an account and are judged more strictly;[15] physicians fill both roles and must be careful never to abuse that authority. Christians, in general, are to "set an example for the believers in speech, in conduct, in love, in faith and in purity."[16] Whether or not recreational marijuana is legal in a particular jurisdiction, its use is a poor Christian witness.

6. **Good stewardship of the environment according to the creation mandate:**[17] The widespread growth of the marijuana industry, according to scientists, will have a deleterious impact on the environment due to deforestation (when grown on natural land) and excessive demands for water, power, pesticides, and fertilizers.[18]

C. SOCIAL

1. **General:** Citizens of a country should consider the known and potential harmful effects of recreational marijuana on individuals and society. Experiences with the harms associated with opioids, alcohol, and tobacco are relevant to the consideration of legalization of recreational marijuana use.

2. **Low-income areas may suffer disproportionately with marijuana legalization:** Recreational marijuana became available in licensed stores in Colorado in 2014.[19] The vast majority of marijuana businesses in Denver service low-income minority neighborhoods.[20] In Colorado, 20 percent of people with incomes under $25,000 consumed marijuana or THC products in 2014, while only 11 percent of those earning over $50,000 consumed the same products.[21]

3. **Increased accidents and deaths:** Between 2013 and 2016 in Colorado, the number of drivers involved in fatal crashes increased 40 percent, and the number of drivers who tested positive for marijuana use increased 145 percent. The prevalence of testing drivers for marijuana use did not change significantly during that time.[22] According to the Colorado Department of Transportation, the number of fatalities with drivers testing positive for 5ng or greater THC decreased from 2016 to 2017.[23] However, state law does not require coroners to test deceased drivers for THC, and not all perform the test. In addition, many police agencies do not test surviving drivers for THC if he or she has already failed a simpler alcohol breath test, thus failing to document drivers who are impaired by both THC and alcohol.[22] Marijuana deaths and injuries have increased in Colorado as marijuana was named as the culprit in fatal fires, explosions, and suicides.[21]

4. **Legalization leads to increased use and abuse, including among minors:** All states with legal recreational marijuana had prior legalization of medical marijuana (see Table at the end of the statement).[24] Evidence suggests that overall availability (whether from medical or recreational marijuana legalization) may lead to an increase in recreational usage among adults and minors. Examples:

   a. One nationwide study found that medical marijuana laws are associated with "increased prevalence of illicit cannabis use and cannabis use disorders" among adults.[25] Marijuana use among those aged 18 to 25 is increasing in states where marijuana is legal.[21]

   b. States with legal marijuana have youth rates that surpass those in states that do not.[21] Colorado's first-time marijuana use among youth leads the nation, with a 65 percent increase since legalization.[21]

   c. Communities with marijuana businesses have greater marijuana use rates among minors. One study from Oregon suggest that communities with a greater number of medical marijuana patients and licensed growers was associated with a higher prevalence of marijuana use among youth from 2006 to 2015. The authors suggest that changing community attitudes in these areas could be influential in teen behavior as well.[26] There is some evidence that 11th graders, but not 8th graders, in Oregon have a higher marijuana use rate in communities without retail bans than in communities with bans.[27]

    d. In Anchorage, where marijuana was legalized in 2015, school suspensions for cannabis use and possession have increased more than 141 percent from 2015 (when legalization was employed) to 2017.[21]

    e. In both Washington and Oregon, recreational marijuana retailers have been cited for selling marijuana to minors.[21]

5. **Commercialization and social media:** Individuals, small businesses, and corporations who profit from marijuana sales are looking to increase its usage. To this end, a variety of advertising venues, including social media platforms, are being used; advertising distortions regarding the benefits of marijuana are not uncommon. When advertisements or staff at marijuana dispensaries or retail stores imply benefits and/or safety (that may not be realistic), people may be enticed to use it. For example, in one cross-sectional study in Colorado, almost 70% of contacted marijuana dispensaries recommended cannabis products to treat nausea during pregnancy,[28] in spite of data suggesting potential harm to fetuses.[1,29-33] Another study examined the website marketing practices of medical and recreational marijuana dispensaries across the U.S., finding that only a few advised about side effects and contraindications. 75% did not include age verification, making products available to youth with convenient online ordering.[34] Exposure to medical marijuana advertising has been associated with greater marijuana use in minors.[35] Physicians should warn their patients about false advertising and the hype on social media.

6. **Opioid addiction:** There has been much hype about marijuana legalization providing a safer replacement for opioid use, with the potential to reduce opioid addiction and overdoses. Evidence is conflicting as to whether this is, in fact, the case,[36] and caution must be used in looking at studies in this area because of bias,[37] unreliability of self-reported use of drugs, the uncertainty of inferring individual substitution behaviors from state-level data relating marijuana legislation and opioid death rates,[38] and other methodological problems. Because societal attitudes may have changed prior to either medical or recreational legalization[26] and because opioid addiction is a complex issue with multiple antecedents that might represent events coinciding with marijuana legalization, it is difficult to define the associations of legalization of marijuana and opioid use. Samples of research:

    a. There are reports that opioid use has increased, rather than decreased, in states legalizing marijuana. In Colorado, for example, opioid use

more than doubled among 10 to 19 year-olds after recreational legalization of marijuana.[21]

b.   Legalization of marijuana in Colorado is associated with short-term
reductions in opioid-related deaths.[39]

c.   Medical legalization appears to be associated with "reductions in
both prescriptions and dosages of Schedule III (but not Schedule II)
opioids received by Medicaid enrollees."[40]

d.   A study that examined opioid use in patients following musculoskeletal trauma found that self-reported marijuana use during recovery
was associated with an increased amount and duration of opioid use.
However, many patients in this study had misperceptions that their
marijuana use reduced both their pain and the amount of opioids
used.[41]

e.   Not only marijuana use but also use of alcohol, illegal methadone,
and other opioids was found to increase in pregnant women after legalization of recreational marijuana in Washington State.[42] Cannabis
use was associated with an increased risk of developing nonmedical
prescription opioid use and opioid use disorder.[43]

7.   **Crime:** Property crimes have increased in Colorado, Alaska, and Oregon
since legalization of recreational marijuana.[21] Black market activity has also
increased post-legalization, as documented in both Colorado and Oregon;
legalization makes illegal marijuana crops easier to conceal. Some of the
illegal operations have been found in national forests or other environmen-
tally-protected areas, and damage has resulted in these areas.[21]

8.   **Profits over people:** The emphasis on marijuana benefits in the form of
excise taxes, job creation, and corporate profits represents a misguided effort
to place profits over the well-being of society and individuals. In addition,
the cost to society of state regulation, law enforcement, accidents, additional
health care costs, high school dropouts, juvenile use, employer-related costs,
and addiction programs will be substantial.[21,44] One report found that "for
every dollar gained in tax revenue, Coloradans spend approximately $4.50
to mitigate the effects of legalization."[44]

9.   **Environmental problems:** Commercial production of marijuana is fraught
with environmental concerns. Marijuana requires a comparatively large
amount of water[45] a yield of 130 bushels/acre, water requirements of 3000
gallons per bushel, and a growing season of 60 days (estimates to err on
the side of the highest water needs per plant and nutrients. Its cultiva-

tion is associated with land clearing, erosion, surface water diversion, use of polluting pesticides and fertilizers, and wildlife poaching.[18] When grown indoors, marijuana requires large amounts of energy[21] with "potentially negative effects on climate."[18] Growing marijuana consumed 1% of the nation's electricity in 2012, which is six times the amount of power used by the entire U.S. pharmaceutical industry. Since then, marijuana cultivation has increased dramatically.[21] The marijuana industry produced almost 400,000 pounds of CO_2 emissions in 2016.[44] A majority of the marijuana consumed in the United States is grown in California, primarily outdoors. There, illegal marijuana production thrives "in sensitive watersheds…which represent habitats for several rare state- and federally listed species," and resulting environmental damage has been documented.[18]

D. MEDICAL

1. **Studies:** Because marijuana has been illegal in the United States until its recent, selective legalization in multiple states, and because it remains illegal federally, high-quality research regarding the safety or risks associated with current recreationally-used marijuana products (especially those containing high levels of THC) is sparse. Studies of recreational products are largely limited to self-reported use and surveys of behaviors. There are large gaps in current knowledge regarding potential risks, and most of the information is in the form of correlations without a clear understanding of causation. It is uncertain whether the potential harms are a function of THC dose or levels in the body and/or of the amounts of other plant compounds or contaminants. In spite of these difficulties, useful information about recreational use of marijuana can be gleaned from research into medical uses as well as from self-report-type studies of recreational use. Prior to presenting such findings, an outline of problems with the research in this area includes:

   a. *Poor reliability:* The research itself has significant problems which limit its reliability. These include factors such as heterogeneity in the active ingredients and contaminants, lack of standard dosing, inadequate research into effects of highly potent types, and variability in the route of consuming marijuana. As an example of the latter, alterations in the number of puffs or volume inhaled may change with the potency of THC in the marijuana being smoked.[46] It is important to note the nature of marijuana derivatives used in any studies—the THC level, delivery method, and quantity. For example, self-reported amount of smoking provides poor data compared to use of FDA-approved standard-dose pharmaceuticals. Conclusive studies can only be done with FDA-regulated medications or pharmaceutical-grade compounds, but such products are less commonly used recreationally.

b. *Insufficient data:* There is a lack of studies on the safety, efficacy, and short-term and long-term effects of marijuana, especially the high potency forms. There are also insufficient studies on the potential drug interactions between cannabis compounds and prescription and non-prescription medications.

c. *Impediments:* Researcher bias; difficulty with achieving double-blind-ed studies; and obtaining properly controlled, adequately-sized, rep-resentative samples are among the methodological problems that may be anticipated in this research area.

d. *Ethical issues:* Adverse health effects of marijuana, especially use of high potency variants and smoking as the means of consumption, highlight ethical problems in exposing research subjects to harm when trying to document the safety or harm of specific consumer products.

e. *Caution:* Weak or absent evidence about harmful effects of marijuana does not mean they do not exist; caution should be used when even limited evidence suggests a possibility of harm.

2. **Medical complications of marijuana use:** Despite the problems with re-search in this area, some of the short-term and long-term effects of mar-ijuana use are being uncovered. In all associations of marijuana use and health complications listed below, the quality of the evidence behind the conclusions is included when available. In the face of insufficient good qual-ity data and conflicting data for some consequences of marijuana use, there may be harmful sequelae that exist but will not be fully elucidated until further research (especially long-term studies) is completed. The lack of current quality research on commonly used recreational marijuana prod-ucts, especially highly potent THC substances, does not mean risk is ab-sent. On the contrary, there is moderate to substantial evidence of health hazards with marijuana use, as listed below. Future research will be needed to provide more definitive answers to questions about effects of recreational marijuana use, and there is potential to find even more harm associated with higher level THC products.

a. *Cancer:* There is limited evidence of a statistical association between current, frequent, or chronic cannabis smoking and one type of tes-ticular tumor, but not current sufficient evidence of associations be-tween marijuana use and other cancer types in adults. There is mini-mal evidence that cannabis use during pregnancy is associated with a greater risk of cancer in offspring.[1]

b. *Respiratory diseases:* There is substantial evidence of an association between chronic marijuana smoking and chronic bronchitis and worsening respiratory symptoms.[47] There is more limited evidence of an association with chronic obstructive pulmonary disease (COPD).[1]

c. *Injury and death:* Substantial evidence correlates cannabis use and increased risk of motor vehicle crashes.[1] Among pediatric populations where cannabis use is legal, there is moderate evidence of increased risk of overdose injuries and respiratory distress.[1]

d. *Pre-and perinatal exposure to maternal cannabis use:* Use of marijuana during pregnancy increased in Washington State after legalization,[42] and is on the rise nationally.[29] Marijuana has potentially serious effects on the developing fetus.[29,30,33] A recent study documented that prenatal THC exposure adversely affects infant neurobehavior and child development up through the teen years,[32] but other researchers feel data is lacking to draw conclusions about long-term effects.[1] Overall review of current studies suggests a substantial association between maternal smoking of marijuana with lower birth weight babies and more limited evidence of a correlation with pregnancy complications for the mother and admission of the newborn to intensive care.[1]

e. *Teen use:* Heavy marijuana use may damage brain development in youth ages 13 to 18. There is evidence of an association between cannabis use and loss of concentration and memory, jumbled thinking, schizophrenia, and early onset paranoid psychosis.[48,49]

f. *Psychosocial impairment:* Moderate evidence correlates acute cannabis use with impaired learning, memory, and attention, and more limited evidence suggests that such impairments may be neurotoxic in that effects are sustained even after prolonged abstinence from cannabis use.[1,50,51] More limited associations exist between cannabis use and impaired academic achievement and outcomes, higher unemployment, lower income, and impaired social functioning.[1] Neurocognitive effects also include a decline in IQ, memory problems, and attentional impairments.[50,51]

g. *Mental health:* There is substantial evidence of statistical association between cannabis use and the development of schizophrenia and other psychoses,[49] with greater risk occurring among more frequent users.[1] In two studies of patients with drug-induced psychosis (most or all being cannabis as the inciting drug), one-third to one-half of the patients later developed a schizophrenia-spectrum disorder.[52,53] Those with drug-induced psychosis were equally as violent as schizophrenia patients who misused drugs.[52] Moderate evidence associates cannabis use with increased incidence of developing depression; suicidal ideation, attempts, and completion; and social anxiety disorder. More limited evidence links cannabis use with certain increased symptoms (e.g. hallucinations) in psychotic disorders, development of bipolar disorder, the development and/or increased symptoms of anxiety disorders, and increased symptoms of posttraumatic stress disorder.[1]

h. *High doses or use of some high potency and/or synthetic cannabis derivatives have produced the following effects:* psychosis, mood alterations, panic attacks, cognitive impairment, dizziness, cardiovascular effects (tachycardia, hypertension, palpitations), nausea, appetite changes, and others.[2] Mental impairment and distressing emotional states, such as paranoia, hallucinations, and psychosis, have caused people to harm themselves and others.[52,54,55]

i. *Addiction:* Use of marijuana can become problematic (marijuana use disorder) which may progress to addiction in some cases; when a person cannot stop using the drug despite interference with many aspects of daily life, use disorder is classified as addiction.[2] A 2015 study suggests that "30 percent of those who use marijuana may have some degree of marijuana use disorder."[2] Marijuana use disorder is frequently "associated with dependence—in which a person feels withdrawal symptoms when not taking the drug."[2] A user may be dependent but not be addicted. Studies estimate that 9 percent of adults[56] and 17 percent of teens who use marijuana will become dependent on it.[2] In 2015 roughly 4 million people in the US were found to have a marijuana use disorder, and 138,000 sought treatment.[2] In the same year in the Netherlands, more first-time entrants and more people overall entered treatment programs for cannabis use than for any other drug.[4] Although modulation of smoking technique may partially blunt the effect of use of high potency cannabis,[46] there is evidence that higher potency marijuana use is associated with increased severity of cannabis dependence.[57] There is moderate evidence of an association between cannabis use and the development of substance dependence and/ or a substance abuse disorder for other substances, including tobacco, alcohol, and illegal drugs.[1,58]

j. *Delivery method:* Smoked substances contain carcinogens and other harmful materials which are known to produce adverse effects on the lungs and other tissues. Marijuana joints may contain "particulate matter, toxic gases, reactive oxygen species, and polycyclic aromatic hydrocarbons at a concentration possibly 20 times that of tobacco smoke."[59] Histopathologic changes in bronchial inflammation that are similar to changes seen with smoking tobacco have been found in marijuana smokers.[59]

E. LEGAL

When recreational marijuana is legally allowed, the state has usually agreed to decriminalize,[60] rather than criminal offense. The offender usually must pay a fine and sometimes is required to take a class on drug abuse. After multiple civil infractions, some states make possession a criminal offense. (Hill KP. Marijuana : The Unbiased Truth About the World's Most Popular Weed. Center City, Minnesota: Hazelden Publishing; 2015. legalize, and regulate the sale of marijuana. In most states, this means that a limited amount of marijuana (intended for personal use) can be purchased at a regulated dispensary by anyone who is 21 years or older with valid government-issued identification. A common limit to the amount of marijuana that can be purchased in states that have legalized marijuana is one ounce.[61] This "small" amount of marijuana is actually enough to make over 50 "joints" and represents an amount a dealer may carry.[62,63] As of late 2018, the District of Columbia and ten states have approved recreational marijuana (see Table below) although the United States still classifies marijuana in the same category as heroin, as a Schedule I Drug, which has "no currently accepted medical use and a high potential for abuse."[64]

F. CMDA RECOMMENDATIONS FOR THE CHRISTIAN HEALTHCARE PROFESSIONAL

1. Because of the health hazards and social ramifications of recreational marijuana use, CMDA does not support its legalization.

2. Because of the adverse health ramifications of marijuana use, and to provide a role model for the community that respects the Biblical principles in section B, healthcare professionals should abstain from using recreational marijuana. They should strongly advise their patients against the use of recreational marijuana, especially minors and pregnant women, due to potential harmful effects.

G. CMDA RECOMMENDATIONS FOR THE CHRISTIAN COMMUNITY

1. Because of the health hazards and social ramifications of recreational marijuana use, CMDA does not support its legalization.

2. Because of the adverse health ramifications of marijuana use, and to provide a role model for the community that respects the Biblical principles in section B, Christians should abstain from using recreational marijuana.

Approved by the Board of Trustees – February 20, 2019

Table: State Recreational Marijuana Laws

States Legalizing Recreational Marijuana	Year Passed	Year Medical Marijuana Legalized
Alaska	2014	1998
California	2016	2000
Colorado	2012 (Retail stores open 2014)	2000
District of Columbia	2014	1998
Maine	2016 (Moratorium on implementing retail sales until 2018)	1999
Massachusetts	2016	2012
Michigan	2018	2008
Nevada	2016	2000
Oregon	2014	1998
Vermont	2018 (limited—no legal production or sales; only allows possession of up to 1 oz. Public consumption illegal)	2004
Washington	2012	1998

(adapted from: *http://www.ncsl.org/research/health/state-medical-marijuana-laws. aspx* and *http://www.ncsl.org/research/civil-and-criminal-justice/marijuana-overview.aspx*)

REFERENCES AND ENDNOTES

1   National Academies of Sciences Engineering and Medicine. The Health Effects of Cannabis and Cannabinoids: The Current State of Evidence and Recommendations for Research. Washington, DC: The National Academies Press; 2017.

2   National Institute on Drug Abuse. Marijuana. June 2018. *https://d14rmgtrwzf5a. cloudfront.net/sites/default/files/1380-marijuana.pdf.*

3   Cort B. Weed, Inc. : The Truth About THC, The Pot Lobby, and the Commercial Marijuana Industry. Deerfield Beach, Florida: Health Communications, Inc.; 2017.

4   European Monitoring Centre for Drugs and Drug Addiction. Netherlands Country Drug Report 2017. Luxembourg: Publications Office of the European Union; 2017.

5   Genesis 1:28

6   Genesis 3

7   Matthew 22:36-40

8   1 Cor. 6:12

9   Deut. 20:3

10 Mark 12:29-30

11 Galatians 5:19-21; 1 Timothy 3:3; Titus 1:7; Eph. 5:18

12 Opioids also may cause an altered state of mind, but relief of severe pain may still dictate their prescription for short term use. Studies are equivocal on marijuana use and

pain; the discussion here is apropos to recreational use, not medical use.

13 Romans 13

14 Daniel 3

15 Hebrews 13:17 and James 3:1

16 1 Timothy 4:12

17 Genesis 1:28

18 Carah JK, Howard JK, Thompson SE, et al. High Time for Conservation: Adding the Environment to the Debate on Marijuana Liberalization. Bioscience 2015; 65(8): 822-9.

19 Ingold J. Colorado Marijuana Guide: 64 of your questions answered. Denver Post. Dec. 31, 2013; updated Feb. 16, 2016. *https://www.thecannabist.co/2013/12/31/colorado-marijuana-guide-64-answers-commonly-asked-questions/1673/.*

20 Migoya D, Baca R. Denver's pot businesses mostly in low-income, minority neighborhoods. The Denver Post. orig. pub. Jan. 2, 2016 updated Jan. 23, 2017.

21 Smart Approaches to Marijuana. Lessons Learned From Marijuana Legalization, 2018. *https://learnaboutsam.org/wp-content/uploads/2018/07/SAM-Lessons-Learned-From-Marijuana-Legalization-Digital-1.pdf.*

22 Migoya D. Exclusive: Traffic fatalities linked to marijuana are up sharply in Colorado. Is legalization to blame? The Denver Post. Orig. pub. Aug. 25, 2017 Updated Dec. 28, 2018.

23 Colorado Department of Transportation. Drugged Driving Statistics: Cannabis-Involved Fatalities in Colorado. *https://www.codot.gov/safety/alcohol-and-impaired-driving/druggeddriving/safety/alcohol-and-impaired-driving/druggeddriving/statistics* (accessed Jan. 9 2019).

24 National Conference of State Legislatures. State Medical Marijuana Laws. 1/23/2019. *http://www.ncsl.org/research/health/state-medical-marijuana-laws.aspx* (accessed Feb. 3 2019).

25 Hasin DS, Sarvet AL, Cerda M, et al. US Adult Illicit Cannabis Use, Cannabis Use Disorder, and Medical Marijuana Laws 1991-1992 to 2012-2013. JAMA Psychiatry 2017; 74(6): 579-88.

26 Paschall MJ, Grube JW, Biglan A. Medical marijuana legalization and marijuana use among youth in Oregon. The Journal of Primary Prevention 2017; 38(3): 329-41.

27 Hatch A. Researchers Tracking Public Health Impacts of Marijuana Legalization. April 14, 2017. *https://nursing.wsu.edu/2017/04/14/13255/* (accessed Feb. 10 2019).

28 Dickson B, Mansfield C, Guiahi M, et al. Recommendations From Cannabis Dispensaries About First-Trimester Cannabis Use. Obstetrics & Gynecology 2018; 131(6): 1031-8.

29 Adashi EY. Brief Commentary: Marijuana Use During Gestation and Lactation—Harmful Until Proved Safe Marijuana Use During Gestation and Lactation. Annals of Internal Medicine 2019; 170(2): 122-.

30 Grant KS, Petroff R, Isoherranen N, Stella N, Burbacher TM. Cannabis use during pregnancy: Pharmacokinetics and effects on child development. Pharmacol Ther 2018; 182: 133-51.

31 Huizink AC. Prenatal cannabis exposure and infant outcomes: overview of studies. Prog Neuropsychopharmacol Biol Psychiatry 2014; 52: 45-52.

32 Jansson LM, Jordan CJ, Velez ML. Perinatal Marijuana Use and the Developing

Child. JAMA: Journal of the American Medical Association 2018; 320(6): 545-6.

33 Volkow ND, Compton WM, Wargo EM. The Risks of Marijuana Use During Pregnancy. JAMA 2017; 317(2): 129-30.

34 Cavazos-Rehg PA, Krauss MJ, Cahn E, et al. Marijuana Promotion Online: an Investigation of Dispensary Practices. Prev Sci 2018.

35 D'Amico EJ, Rodriguez A, Tucker JS, Pedersen ER, Shih RA, D'Amico EJ. Planting the seed for marijuana use: Changes in exposure to medical marijuana advertising and subsequent adolescent marijuana use, cognitions, and consequences over seven years. Drug & Alcohol Dependence 2018; 188: 385-91.

36 National Institute on Drug Abuse. What is medical marijuana? June 2018 June 2018. *https://www.drugabuse.gov/publications/drugfacts/marijuana-medicine* (accessed February 5 2019).

37 Example of bias: An article by Lucas (Lucas P. Rationale for cannabis-based interventions in the opioid overdose crisis. Harm Reduction Journal 2017; 14: 1-6) advocated for medical and recreational legalization of marijuana as a way to reduce opioid addiction and overdoses. However, the Methods section did not reveal the mechanism of article selection nor any other methods, no conflicting data was mentioned at all, and the author's conflict of interest was noted in small print at the end of the article—he is VP and stockholder with a federally authorized medical cannabis production & research company in Canada.

38 Caputi TL, Sabet KA. Population-level analyses cannot tell us anything about individual-level marijuana-opioid substitution. American Journal of Public Health 2018; 108(3): e12-e.

39 Livingston MD, Barnett TE, Delcher C, Wagenaar AC. Recreational Cannabis Legalization and Opioid-Related Deaths in Colorado, 2000-2015. American Journal of Public Health 2017; 107(11): 1827-9.

40 Liang D, Bao Y, Wallace M, Grant I, Shi Y. Medical cannabis legalization and opioid prescriptions: evidence on US Medicaid enrollees during 1993-2014. Addiction 2018; 113(11): 2060-70.

41 Bhashyam AR, Heng M, Harris MB, Vrahas MS, Weaver MJ. Self-Reported Marijuana Use Is Associated with Increased Use of Prescription Opioids Following Traumatic Musculoskeletal Injury. J Bone Joint Surg Am 2018; 100(24): 2095-102.

42 Grant TM, Graham JC, Carlini BH, Ernst CC, Brown NN. Use of marijuana and other substances among pregnant and parenting women with substance use disorders: Changes in Washington state after marijuana legalization. Journal of Studies on Alcohol and Drugs 2018; 79(1): 88-95.

43 Olfson M, Wall MM, Shang-Min L, Blanco C. Cannabis Use and Risk of Prescription Opioid Use Disorder in the United States. American Journal of Psychiatry 2018; 175(1): 47-53.

44 Centennial Institute. Economic and Social Costs of Legalized Marijuana: Colorado Christian University, 2018.

45 Marijuana requires more water for growth than many other plants. It takes about 22 liters of water a day per marijuana plant in northern CA. (Carah JK, Howard JK, Thompson SE, et al. High Time for Conservation: Adding the Environment to the Debate on Marijuana Liberalization. Bioscience 2015; 65(8): 822-9.) Another estimate for marijuana is 900 gallons of water per plant per season (*https://www.marijua-*

naventure.com/report-on-water-usage/). Using estimates of 22,000 corn plants/acre, a yield of 130 bushels/acre, water requirements of 3000 gallons per bushel, and a growing season of 60 days (estimates to err on the side of the highest water needs per plant), a corn plant does not require more than18 gallons of water per plant per season, or 1 liter per day. An average adult requires about 2.5 liters of water per day.

46   Pol P, Liebregts N, Brunt T, et al. Cross-sectional and prospective relation of cannabis potency, dosing and smoking behaviour with cannabis dependence: an ecological study. Addiction 2014; 109(7): 1101-9.

47   Tashkin DP. Marijuana and Lung Disease. CHEST 2018; 154(3): 653-63.

48   Dr. Phil Tibbo, one of the leaders in the medical field and initiator of Nova Scotia's Weed Myths campaign targeting teens, has seen firsthand evidence of what heavy use can do as director of Nova Scotia's Early Psychosis Program. His brain research shows that regular marijuana use leads to an increased risk of developing psychosis and schizophrenia, effectively exploding popular and rather blasé notions that marijuana is "harmless" to teens and "recreational use" is simply "fun and healthy." Multiple researchers have all come to the same conclusion: the younger the brain, the worse the effects in both the short-term and long-term. (Tibbo P, Crocker CE, Lam RW, Meyer J, Sareen J, Aitchison KJ. Implications of Cannabis Legalization on Youth and Young Adults. Canadian Journal of Psychiatry 2018; 63(1): 65-71.)

49   Malone DT, Hill MN, Rubino T. Adolescent cannabis use and psychosis: epidemiology and neurodevelopmental models. British Journal of Pharmacology 2010; 160(3): 511-22.

50   Harvey PD. Smoking Cannabis and Acquired Impairments in Cognition: Starting Early Seems Like a Really Bad Idea. Am J Psychiatry 2019; 176(2): 90-1.

51   Morin J-FG, Afzali MH, Bourque J, et al. A Population-Based Analysis of the Relationship Between Substance Use and Adolescent Cognitive Development. American Journal of Psychiatry 2019; 176(2): 98-106.

52   Crebbin K, Mitford E, Paxton R, Turkington D. First-episode drug-induced psychosis: A medium term follow up study reveals a high-risk group. Social Psychiatry and Psychiatric Epidemiology 2009; 44(9): 710-5.

53   Arendt M, Rosenberg R, Foldager L, Perto G, Munk-Jørgensen P. Cannabis-induced psychosis and subsequent schizophrenia-spectrum disorders: Follow-up study of 535 incident cases. The British Journal of Psychiatry 2005; 187(6): 510-5.

54   Korkmaz Sshc, Turhan L, İzci F, Sağlam S, Atmaca M. Sociodemographic and clinical characteristics of patients with violence attempts with psychotic disorders. European Journal of General Medicine 2017; 14(4): 94-8.

55   Douglas KS, Guy LS, Hart SD. Psychosis as a Risk Factor for Violence to Others: A Meta-Analysis. Psychological Bulletin; 2009. p. 679-706.

56   Lopez-Quintero C, Perez de los Cobos J, Hasin DS, et al. Probability and predictors of transition from first use to dependence on nicotine, alcohol, cannabis, and cocaine: Results of the National Epidemiologic Survey on Alcohol and Related Conditions (NESARC). Drug and Alcohol Dependence 2011; 115(1-2): 120-30.

57   Freeman TP, Winstock AR. Examining the profile of high-potency cannabis and its association with severity of cannabis dependence. Psychological Medicine 2015; 45(15): 3181-9.

58   Blanco C, Hasin DS, Wall MM, et al. Cannabis use and risk of psychiatric disorders:

Prospective evidence from a US national longitudinal study. JAMA Psychiatry 2016; 73(4): 388-95.

59 Caviedes I, Labarca G, Silva CF, Fernandez-Bussy S. Marijuana Use, Respiratory Symptoms, and Pulmonary Function. Annals of Internal Medicine 2019; 170(2): 142-.

60 Twenty-two states and the District of Columbia have decriminalized small amounts of marijuana. (National Conference of State Legislatures. Marijuana Overview. Dec. 14, 2018. *http://www.ncsl.org/research/civil-and-criminal-justice/marijuana-overview.aspx* (accessed Feb. 10 2019).) This makes possession of a small amount of marijuana (usually an ounce) a civil, rather than criminal offense. The offender usually must pay a fine and sometimes is required to take a class on drug abuse. After multiple civil infractions, some states make possession a criminal offense. (Hill KP. Marijuana : The Unbiased Truth About the World's Most Popular Weed. Center City, Minnesota: Hazelden Publishing; 2015.)

61 Recreational Marijuana Laws by State--Updated. *https://usaweed.org/recreational-marijuana-laws-state/Feb.* 12, 2019).

62 Hill KP. Marijuana : The Unbiased Truth About the World's Most Popular Weed. Center City, Minnesota: Hazelden Publishing; 2015.

63 For more information on pros and cons of decriminalization, see: Hill KP. Marijuana : The Unbiased Truth About the World's Most Popular Weed. Center City, Minnesota: Hazelden Publishing; 2015.

64 DEA. Drug Scheduling. *https://www.dea.gov/drug-scheduling* (accessed Jan. 4, 2019 2019).

ACKNOWLEDGMENTS

DEBTS AND LESSONS[1]

Robert Frost ends his poem, "Two Tramps in Mud Time," with the following lines:

> *My object in living is to unite*
> *My avocation and my vocation*
> *As my two eyes make one in sight.*
> *Only where love and need are one,*
> *And the work is play for mortal stakes,*
> *Is the deed ever really done*
> *For Heaven and the future sakes.*

The setting is a beautiful April day in New England and the narrator in Frost's poem is splitting wood. It's a moment when the rhythm of work (need) connects with the harmonies of nature, love and God. I believe Frost is expressing one of the fundamental insights of faith that there is a mystery—a deeper meaning, a purpose, an eternal ring—to even the mundane things in life.

This book has united my avocation and vocation. It was never meant to be a means to an end, but an end in itself. It is the result of a humble and, if I am honest, flawed and futile search for truth in a world still reeling from The Fall and The First Lie.

This book would not have been possible without the inspiration, encouragement and contributions of an army of people—too many to ever list. I am deeply indebted to each of them for the lessons they have taught me directly or indirectly or from their example.[1]

First, I would like to thank my incredibly devoted and selfless colleagues on the Marijuana subcommittee at Christian Medical & Dental Associations (CMDA) and the American Academy of Medical Ethics (AAME): Margie Shealy, Dr. Sharon Quick, Dr. David Stevens, Dr. Greg Schmedes, Dr. Carley Robinson and Dr. Rick McCain. Thank you for demonstrating passion, integrity, hard work, sacrifice, love, prudence and persistence. I would never have thought about tackling a project like this if we hadn't built the foundation together when serving on the committee and writing the policy statements. Each of you, in reality, are my co-authors.

I'd like to thank every single person at CMDA. It is truly an exceptional organization, and I am profoundly indebted to each and every one of you. When like-minded colleagues were scarce, you were my lifeline these past 41 years. I'd like to especially call out Dr. David Stevens and Dr. Mike Chupp, who both encouraged me and gave their approval for this book. My dear colleague and brother, Dr. David Stevens, asked me to speak at the CMDA National Convention in 2019 (when a book was the last thing on my mind) and Dr. Mike Chupp approved the publication even before officially becoming the new CEO of CMDA. I am deeply grateful to both of them for the privilege and opportunity.

When writing this book, I became even more aware of the tremendous influence my mom and dad had on me when I was young. My mom read to me endlessly and, no matter how tired she was, always took me to the library whenever I asked. There was no sacrifice too great when it came to her children. And my dad encouraged the exploration of new ideas and words constantly. From giving my brothers and me a nickel for every new word we looked up in the dictionary to constantly giving me new books to read and consider, he enlarged my mind, my dreams and my possibilities.

This book would never have been written if I hadn't heard about substance addiction, stigma and marijuana over numerous meals and phone calls with my two winsome, sagacious and irrepressible sons: Jonathan Avery, MD, Director of Addiction Psychiatry at Weil Cornell Medical College, and Joseph Avery, JD, MA, a Columbia Law School graduate and current PhD candidate at Princeton. I especially am indebted to them for the chapter on addiction stigma and their endless encouragement.

I cannot say enough about my youngest child and only daughter, Juli. No matter how busy she was, she always asked me how the book was going in her tender-hearted, grace-filled and compassionate way. Her concerned encouragement always touched my heart and energized my spirit.

And I cannot and will never find enough words to express my love and heartfelt gratitude to my forever-love, Jan. You kept the trains running while I hunkered down in the basement writing and researching. I would never have finished this book without our daily energizing walks, your prayers, love, editing, encouragement and healthy gourmet meals. Your ceaseless and sacrificial love help me daily to see more clearly the heart of God.

Finally, where would I be without my Lord and Savior, Jesus Christ? His faithfulness, kindness and mercy have saved me over and over…from myself. *Soli Deo gloria.*

CITATION

1   Gregory Hays in his translation of *Mediations* (Marcus Aurelius) entitled Book 1, "Debts and Lessons" because "Marcus reflects on what he learned from various individuals in his life, either directly or indirectly or from their example."

ABOUT THE AUTHOR

JAMES ALAN AVERY, MD, CMD, FAAHPM, FCCP, FACP

Dr. Avery is the National Medical Director for Diversicare Healthcare and Visiting Assistant Professor of Medicine at the University of Virginia's School of Medicine. Dr. Avery is a Fellow in the American College of Physicians, the American College of Chest Physicians and the American Academy of Hospice and Palliative Medicine.

He was awarded the Roger Bone Award for National Leadership in End-of-Life Care and the Lillian Wald Award for his work in hospice and palliative medicine in New York City. Dr. Avery was named "One of the 50 Most Influential Physician Executives" by *Modern Physician* magazine and was also nominated as "One of the 100 Most Influential People in Healthcare" by *Modern Healthcare* magazine.

He is the author of the acclaimed children's book *How's the Water, Girls?*

He has been married for almost four decades to his lifelong sweetheart Jan, and they have three adult children (whose names all begin with the letter J: Jonathan, Joseph and Juli) and two grandchildren (Elena and Gabriel). He loves his daughter-in-law Maria and son-in-law Ian as if they were his own. He lives in Charlottesville, Virginia with Jan, two cats and dog Chester.

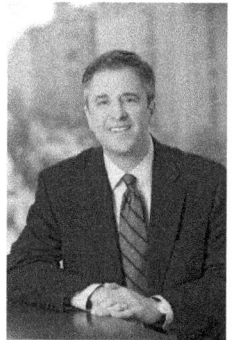

www.ingramcontent.com/pod-product-compliance
Lightning Source LLC
Chambersburg PA
CBHW051715020426
42333CB00014B/1000